Parkinson's Disease
Every Movement's A Dance

Thoughts and Stories of Faith and Parkinson's disease

Copyright 2017

Mark Thorsell

All Rights Reserved

To my wife, Marcia,

At this moment in our life together, we have known each other over half of the time we have spent on this earth. Life has risen far above my expectation. The reason this is true is you. Neither history or eternity will ever have the ability to judge the true value of any one human life. We are the least qualified to judge ourselves. My prayer is that I have loved you close to your expectations.

Table of Contents

Forward	7
Beginnings	15
I Have Joy	24
More Than God	38
Off In The Distance	47
The Pursuit	54
The Third Group	59
A New Table	76
Coping Mechanisms	96
I Dream Of Movement	109
Light Into Darkness	120
The Selfishness Of Sickness	128
Healing In A Fallen World	143
Right Choices Are Hard	156
Different Universes	165
More Like Jesus	182
Microscopic Adversaries	193

Naked	204
In A Heartbeat	216
We Serve At The Pleasure Of The King	226
Words	249
Simply Human	281
Words 2	297
Just Out Of Reach	314
A Strange Question	325
Music And Words	336
Stricken With Parkinson's	357
Not For A Lack Of Stones	374
Cries From Heaven	385

Forward

When my kids were small, they would play music and ask me to dance. This was long before I was diagnosed with Parkinson's disease. I would stand and start this series of contorted movements and they would always laugh, delighted by this spectacle they said no one else could recreate. After my diagnoses, when the Parkinson's started to affect my body, I was walking past my wife in our kitchen and my foot slipped. I started to fall but was able to catch myself. I could see she was concerned. I took her face in my hands and said, "Every movement's a dance."

As I watch my movements and the movements of my fellow Parkinson's brothers and sisters, I don't see them as the result of a lack of dopamine or the side effect of a medication, but as a choreographed dance not completely controlled by the dancer. I would rather think of it that way instead of them being random movements that have no meaning or expression. We may not be able to control our dance most of the time, but for whatever reason, they are a part of us. Everyone says something to the world around them by their movements. Those of us with Parkinson's may just be a little more expressive.

I am a follower of Jesus and I have Parkinson's disease. I see life through the eyes of a Christian man. I move through this world with a body affected by Parkinson's.

Because healing is a large part of my faith, I have had to come to grips with the fact that I am a Christian and I still have Parkinson's. As I wrestle with this, I have found that writing helps me in that process. In this book, I am placing my thoughts and stories. Most of them are about my life and thoughts related to Parkinson's. Some are just stories. Some are from my previous book titled, "With Half My Brain Tied Behind My Back." I reviewed those thoughts and stories and updated and corrected where needed. The rest will either be new or ones I did not include in the previous book.

I want to again include this disclaimer; I am not a writer. I have little education in sentence structure or grammar. I wouldn't know a participle if it was dangling right in front of me. Despite spellcheck, there will be misspelled words. I do my own editing so mistakes will be made. With that in mind, I will try and do my best.

Beginnings

Even when you have more years behind you than are ahead of you, there are beginnings. They become less frequent as the years go by, but they never stop until you stop. Every moment is an opportunity for something new to begin. I have been married for 33 years and raised 3 people. I have worked ever since I was 15. I have lived a life that has risen above my expectations. That doesn't mean the sun has always shined. It has rained. But for some reason the sun has been brighter and it has rained less often than I imagined it would. It's hard to say where the expectations that my life has risen above came from. I just thought when I got here and looked back, I would not have enjoyed my life as much as I have. I feel there are two primary reasons for this.

#1 - I have great parents.

#2 - I found Jesus, (or He found me,) when I was 6 years old.

Because of those two factors, I have been able to make more good choices than bad choices. I don't know why I had the parents I had or why God allowed me to find Him. I don't know why other people have bad parents, or were born someplace where they didn't find God. I do know that we live in a world we created. A better way to say it is, we live in a world we recreated. God created

the world and mankind perfect. A part of that perfection was He gave us the power of choice. When we were confronted with the first choice between right and wrong, we chose poorly. Our choice recreated the world. From the moment we did this, our choices from day to day and moment to moment have set into motion...
disease, hunger, poverty, violence, injustice, perversion, lying,

selfishness and everything else that flies in the face of perfection. We are responsible for all that is wrong in the world. Our bad choice even threw off the balance of nature and the universe. When what we call "a natural disaster" happens and things are broken and people die, the question is asked, "Why would God allow this to happen?" When what should be called "an unnatural disaster" happens, it's our fault, not God's. It's our fault that there is hunger and poverty in the world. Even in this fallen world, we have the resources to meet most people's needs...we just choose not to or turn away.

God is good, all the time. Satan is bad, all the time.

It was up to us which one to choose when the first choice was made.

It's been up to us ever since.

I Have Joy

Life is a journey. Some parts of the journey are interesting and some are not. Even though more and more people are having to walk this Parkinson' life than ever before, most people have no idea what it's like to live this life. I thought that keeping you up to date on any insights I hoped to be able to share would be of some value. I was hoping to learn life lessons that would help me and maybe help other people live happy lives with some kind of challenging condition that won't go away.

I was surprised by how I felt when the doctor told me that I had Parkinson's disease. It was a weird combination of relief, happiness, and freedom. You would expect to feel something like fear or sadness when you are told you have a progressive, degenerative brain disease that there is no cure for. I felt neither of those things.

For some time before the diagnosis, I had not felt good. I had constant pain and a host of unwelcome and uninvited problems with my body and mind. I was suffering. What made it worse was trying to find out why this was happening to me and find a way to make it stop. Being God's child, my fear was that I had done something that caused this to happen to me. Did I let something in the door of my life that gave it the right to do this to me? Or was it something I did to take me out from under God's protection leaving me vulnerable?

My life had not been a perfect life. I do make wrong and stupid decisions from time to time. And I believe like most people, I struggled with repeated sin and haven't always chosen what I knew was right.

When you are saved at 6 years old, I don't think you can say you were a sinner saved by grace. I believe in the age of accountability and when I reached it, I had not yet become a sinner. (I know every person is born into sin because of what our first parents did in Eden. I'm referring to having to be responsible for personal sin).

Every person is responsible for the things they do that are wrong, saved and unsaved. The difference is the unsaved have no way out and are totally subject to the consequences of their actions and at the mercy of the adversary. We that are saved are also responsible for the consequences of our actions, but we have the opportunity to be forgiven, because we have a Father that forgives. Both the saved and unsaved are subject to this fallen world along with being in danger from the trains we willingly lay down in front of. The rain falls on the just and the unjust, the drought also hits them both.

There I was in the parking lot of my doctor, having suffered the last few years and trying the whole time to find out why and correct anything I had done or not done to cause it, not being able to put a name or a face on my tormentors. But now, someone had just given

them a name,
Parkinson's disease.

For some reason, that made me feel better. I still had pain and all the symptoms, but now there was also hope. Hope that there were tools to battle this previously unrecognized foe. Hope that there were people that had the wisdom and knowledge to fight this foe with me.

I am still coming to terms as to the "why I have Parkinson's", but the why doesn't really matter to me anymore. I just believe that God knows what He is doing. It's my job to trust Him, do what I know is right, following his command to love Him and love others.

The path this journey is taking is getting steeper and more difficult to walk. I have lost my ability to work. Many of the things in life that I used to enjoy I no longer care about or I have lost the ability to do. My body is becoming less cooperative and rebellious. But I'm happy!

I have joy. The joy of having the best and most interesting person I have ever known as my wife. The joy of having three children that, if it were possible to choose your children, I wouldn't have even come close to the fantastic ones I got. The joy of bringing into our family the perfect people our children chose to marry. The joy of grandchildren. The joy of having a God that is working endlessly in the most microscopic recesses of my life. The joy of friendship and family, where the line between them becomes blurred. The joy of the anticipation of heaven. I have joy!

More Than God

Christian's get sick.
The first time the words "Parkinson's Disease" were applied to me back in 2009, I started to think about healing. I believe that the supernatural removal of sickness and injury by God is real. I believe that my family and I have been the receivers of supernatural healing. It's like my belief in the other things we thank God for...wisdom, protection, provision, joy and everything else that

I believe God supernaturally gives us. God is active in our lives and cares about us. I also believe His ability to provide these things for us is limited. Limited not by Him, but limited by the fact that man changed God's original universe.

We, mankind, started out perfect. God made us that way. We didn't get sick, we had no lack. Everything was provided for us and it was all good. But we were not satisfied with everything. We wanted more. We wanted something we were not made to have. We wanted something more than God. We wanted something apart from God. We wanted to be God. And when a creature that had wanted the same thing, and had suffered the consequences, offered those things to us, we said yes. From that moment, we have suffered the consequences of wanting more than God and the choice of saying yes to the creature's offer.

But instead of giving up on mankind, God has been working ever since to restore us to our original state of perfection. He desires our restoration so much, that He was willing to sacrifice His Son to achieve it. Everything He has done here on earth and beyond, ever since we believed the lie that there is anything more than God, has been done for our restoration. But even though His act of offering His Son provided the way for mankind to be restored, we have to want to be restored and accept it the way He provided. We still live in a world that offers us more than God, even though those things do not exist. We still live in a world that offers life apart from God. It is an illusion. But we are still given the choice of God or more than God. And most still

choose the illusion.
We, the people that choose God, still have to live in a world that was given away. That is the result of mankind wanting and choosing more than God. We gave it away to the creature that offered us the illusion that there was more than God. God had given the world to man to have dominion, and we gave the right to be here and work here to the creature. Even

though God has provided the way for our restoration to perfection, we are still born and live out our lives in bodies that are made of the same material this fallen earth is made of. And we are subject to the same imperfections. We get sick. We get injured. We are born with flaws. We can find ourselves in a place of not having the basic things we need to live. The whole universe from our bodies to the stars, continually groan for the sons of God to be revealed. That has not happened yet. When it does, we will no longer get sick. Our bodies will never need healing. And we will return to the perfection God originally planned for us. Until then, Christians get sick. It seems like, some get healed, some don't.

Off In The Distance

There I am, off in the distance. I know it's me because of all the years we spent together. I look pretty much the same as I always have, just smaller. Because of the distance, it's hard to hear what I'm saying and it looks like I'm moving in slow motion. Those that are passing me by are trying not to look at me, but I can see their sideways glances when they think I'm not looking. I do see them, but I'm not troubled by them. The truth is, I'm glad they choose to see me. It means I'm still here. There are rare moments when I am afraid they won't look anymore. I'm afraid a time may come when I will look and I won't be there. But these are just moments.

There it is, off in the distance. The world that was once mine. The world used to be a lot bigger and was full of things that were free for the taking. The world is much smaller now and much of what had been free for the taking, things that only required me to reach out and grasp them, are now out of my reach. As the world grew smaller, the distances grew longer. Time slowed down.

There they are, off in the distance.... standing beside me...standing with me. They don't seem to notice I'm different than I used to be. I try not to be different than I used to be, but most of the time it's not up to me. I'm glad they are still there, though there seem to be fewer than before. I guess that's because the world is a lot smaller so there's not as much room as there was before.

There He is, off in the distance...giving me hope and joy...making all my self-perceived challenges fade, and revealing a future of effortless movement that will go on forever. Encouraging me with the knowledge that even though the rest of my journey may be slow and unsteady, once the distance is crossed and I arrive home, what is waiting for me is so wonderful, all of the pain of this life will be forgotten. That's when my true journey begins. My eternal journey with God.

The Pursuit

I am being pursued by a foe that is bent on stealing anything and everything he can from me. But guess what... he's after <u>everyone</u>.
All of us have a dream of what our lives should be like. Mine did not include Parkinson's disease. Of course, I know if it hadn't been that, it would have been something else. He pursues everyone and his goal is to destroy everyone. His mind is fixed on that goal.
The great news is

someone else is pursuing us and He is infinitely more powerful and more tenacious for our good and will ultimately rescue us from the intent of our adversary.

So, while I (and we) must endure the pokes and scratches from this toothless and declawed tiger, a time will come when he will be exposed for what he really is by the One who made us and keeps us every day. Yes, I am getting tired and probably will continue to lose abilities and my body will continue to be subject to the inconveniences caused by living in this fallen world. Fortunately, I have all of you to cheer me on and I know the One who helps me move, despite my lack of dopamine. Plus, I am so blest....I have a GREAT wife who constantly fills the voids that continuously open up in our lives due to my Parkinson's....Great kids and mates and grandkids that are a constant flow of joy and challenges.

Life is good. God is Great, all the time!

The Third Group

Despite the differences in appearance, hair color…. eye color…. skin color…. male or female, we are all born the same. We are simply human, not a part of a group or tribe or color or anything else, nothing that would distinguish us from any other human that has ever lived or will ever live. Anything that labels us was put there by ourselves or someone else. The truest connection we all have is that we are all born lost. The only thing that really matters is will we remain lost.

We will all die.

After we are dead, we will all stand before God. Everyone. The place where we will stand will be flat and level. There will be no status or position or labels. We will all be the same.

We will all be asked one

question. It will not be one of these;

What did you eat or what did you refrain from eating?
What did you touch or what did you avoid touching?
What did you do or what didn't you do?
What group were you a part of?

The question that will be asked will be, "Did you believe Jesus?"

If the answer is yes, the reason it's yes will not be because of anything done or not done during our life…except for one thing. Did we believe Him and what He did?

There is a question that could be asked, but won't be asked. "What evidence can be offered to prove your belief in Jesus?" If the question was asked, the answer would be "None." But the question won't be asked.

Evidence will not be presented. If evidence were to be allowed to be presented, it would not include eating this or not eating that, doing this good thing or doing that bad thing. It could include a life of loving God with everything. A life of loving others more than loving ourselves.

I believe that one of the

gifts God gave everyone through Jesus was freedom and simplicity. In all my years of knowing Jesus, the truth is, for myself and many others I have met along the way, trying to figure out what God wants to say to me, "Me", has been a challenge that kept me in a place of frustration and confusion for a long time.

Then I realized something. God's desire and expectation for

everyone is to know Him and His Son. He would not have made it hard to do this. He would not expect this of us and desire this of us and then hide. He gave us a book that we could hold in our hands and understand. He wanted to tell us where we have been, where we are now and where we are going.

I'm still somewhat puzzled about where we have been and why He did some of the things

he did and the way he did them. I'm pretty clear on where we are now and I do know where I'm going.
For the where we came from, I just need to trust Him to help me understand the things that I need to understand.
For the where we are now, I'm thankful to Him for the Holy Spirit that speaks to my spirit the deep mysteries and the simple truths of living a life for God and for

other people. And as for knowing where I'm going, I'm thankful to Jesus for providing the way and the assurance of it.

I do understand that God would have wanted us to have made different choices, starting with our first parents saying no to the serpents offer. But they said yes. And even though they said yes, God still loved us. He loved us enough to provide a way for all of us to be able to come to a point in our lives where we have the opportunity to choose Him over something else, the same offer our first parents were given. And we are free to make the choice.

God's plan has always been the same, to win us back…to save us from making the wrong choice. The bible is the story of Him doing that. It is a story with many different parts that take place over thousands of years. Much of the story applies to me directly and much of it applies to me indirectly.

This is what the bible story is;

Once upon a time, God created everything. He created a man and a woman. The man and woman had the ability to make a choice. To choose between God or something else. They chose something else. That choice separated the man and woman from God. The man and woman were now lost. All their children would be born lost. But God wanted them back. So, He made a way back. It would take a long time and the journey would be costly. So costly, that it would mean the death of His Son. But God loved us so much, He was willing to pay the price. God's willingness to do this gave every man the right to make the choice between God and something else. Everyone has the opportunity to make the choice. Hopefully a better choice than our first parents made. During the journey from our first parents until this moment, God has been working at restoring us to Him. He separated groups of people from each other by language and color. He made rules for men to follow for protection and direction until they were no longer needed. He sent his Son to restore us to Himself. He sent us a counselor to show us how to love and live.

And he has prepared a perfect place for us to be with Him and each other forever.

What gives us the right to enter this place is not who we are or what we have or haven't done or how much we had or didn't have. The right is a gift freely given simply by loving God and His Son and living a life that shows it, and by loving others more than ourselves and living a life that shows it. Everyone that tries to add extra requirements for entry into this perfect place are wasting their time. Everyone that tries to earn the right to enter by what they do or refrain from doing will remain lost forever without God.

That's simply the Bible's

story.

So, when God asks us the only question we will be asked to answer, what will our answer be?
Remember, it will be a yes or no question.

A New Table

My name is Demikus. I am a citizen of Rome. I was born in Rome. I have lived here all my life. And I am a carpenter. I make furniture. I'm pretty good at it, if I do say so myself. My wife's name was Salara. She died 4 years ago giving birth to our only child, our son and my joy, Justic. He was born with a body and mind that, though beautiful, do not function for him. He rarely moves, and when he does, his movements are slow and contorted. His eyes, though deep blue like a clear summer sky, have never seen me or shown any sign of recognition of anything. When his eyes are open, he just stares blankly past me. Except for a few and infrequent low groans or moans, I have never heard his voice. I love him with more than all my heart. He is a constant joy for me and a never-ending reminder of the love of my life, who gave her life so my son could live.

Ever since the moment he came into the world, we have never been apart. He is always with me. When he was small, I would carry my tool box in one hand and Justic in his basket in the other. Now that he's 4, when I go out to work, I carry him on my back, in a pack I made for him. My neighbors and my customers now think of us as one person. Where I go, he goes. I think he is happy. I guess I choose to believe he is happy.

A man came to Rome about a year ago. He arrived under guard and moved, or a better way to say it, was put into a house across the city and has remained there ever since. He is not allowed to leave and the house is continually guarded. I have heard he is allowed to have people in and his friends are allowed to meet his needs, but he never leaves the house. There are many rumors about who he is, (or was). Some say he was a powerful Roman official that got on the wrong side of Caesar. Others say he got on the wrong side of some Jewish leaders. Who knows? Anyway, it's none of my business. That's what I thought anyway, until last week.

A man I had never seen before came to my house the Monday before last. He said he had a job for me. His friend needed a table. The table he had was not large enough for him to work on. I asked the man what kind of work his friend did. He said he was a writer. He told me the size of table he needed, I told him the price I would charge, and he agreed. He told me the location of the house where I would be delivering the table, paid the deposit, and asked when I would have it finished. I told him a week and he nodded his head in approval and left.

So, for the next week, Justic and I worked on the table. Measuring, cutting, fitting, sanding. I would do the physical work, and my son would be by my side, encouraging me. When the table was finished, I tied the pieces on my pull cart, loaded my tools and set Justic in his pack and carefully placed him on my back. I took hold of the pull poles on the front of my cart and my son and I started our trip to the customers house.

As we approached the location the man had indicated, I asked a group of people sitting at a cafe if they could tell me where the house was that matched my description. A short time later, we came to the house. I was surprised to see two soldiers guarding the front door. As we approached the door, one of the guards asked me to state my business. Right when I was about to answer, the man that had ordered the table came out the front door and explained my business to the guards. They moved away from the door so Justic and I could carry the new table inside. After being shown where the table was to be assembled, we brought it in and put it in its place. When we were finished, the man paid us. As we were about to leave, the man said the person that I had built the table for would like to speak to me, if I had the time. I agreed and he directed me to some stairs he told me led to a terrace where I would find him. We climbed the stairs and came to a bright and open terrace. There was a man sitting on a chair in the middle of the space with his back to us. As we approached, he rose from the chair with substantial effort and turned towards us. He was very old and had snow white hair. His face was cracked and wrinkled and marked with much more than age. But in the center of this ravaged face were two eyes I have a hard time describing even now. They seemed to pierce straight into my heart. They showed so much wisdom, strength, compassion, pain and heartbreak, I could hardly look into them. He offered his hand. I grasped it. It was even more twisted and scared than his face, but steady and strong. He said, "I have been so wanting to meet the two of you." Most people only address me, and ignore Justic. I told him, this is my son, Justic, and I'm Demikus. He said, "My name is Paul". There was another chair in the corner of the terrace. He pulled it out and placed it next to the one he had been sitting in and asked, "Would you mind if we sat and talked for a while?" I told him that I wouldn't mind and prepared to bring my son around to my lap so I could sit down. But before I got him settled, Paul asked, " Would you mind if I hold him while we talk?" Taken by surprise, because no one had ever asked that of me before, I hesitated for a moment, but then handed my precious son to a man I had just met. He gently cradled Justic in his arms, and as we talked, he would slowly rock him back and forth. We talked for about an hour. I told him about my growing up in Rome and learning to be a carpenter. He told me his best friend is a carpenter. I told him how hard it was losing my wife and what a joy Justic was in my life. He told me stories about all the places he had been and even being shipwrecked at sea more than once. It started getting late, so I told him we had better start for home. With that he gave my son a kiss on his forehead. He gave him a last gentle hug before handing my sleeping boy back to me. We said goodbye and as I approached the top step to go down, I turned and the old man smiled.

Justic slept all the way home. When we arrived, it was late. I placed him carefully in his bed and he stayed asleep.

The next morning as the sun rose in my window and its rays rested on my face, a shadow moved across the light for a moment. I sprang to my feet to see who was in my room. I saw a small figure standing, looking out the window. As my eyes focused, I discovered it was my son! I ran over to him and embraced him. I turned him around so I could look at his face. He was smiling and for the first time I saw him in his eyes. As I cried, he hugged me like he was trying to comfort me. The whole time he was smiling. Was this real or a dream. I took a couple steps back and he followed me. A bird landed on the windowsill and chirped. Justic turned towards the window, pointed his finger at the bird, and also for the first time laughed. This was no dream. My precious son was well. I spent the next few hours watching him and playing with him. We went to all our neighbors and I introduced them to my son. All they had ever seen was the way he used to be and everyone was amazed and asked how this could be. I told them I had no idea. But I thought to myself, I do have an idea. That afternoon, Justic and I started out to see Paul again. I had to find out what had happened. Somehow, he had given me my son. And as we traveled, rather than riding on my back in silence, I felt my son's

hand in mine and heard
his laughter as we
walked together.

Coping Mechanisms

I have Parkinson's disease because my brain no longer produces a chemical called dopamine. My body needs this chemical to move and function correctly. My brain can no longer produce dopamine due to the fact that the cells that make it are dying. It may be 10 to 20 years after they start to die that a person will notice any significant symptoms. There is no test a doctor can do to diagnose Parkinson's disease. It is a symptom diagnosed condition. When I saw the neurologist in 2009, I was referred to him by my family doctor after I described some things I had noticed going wrong. The neurologist spent about 30 minutes asking me questions and having me move different parts of my body. When the 30 minutes were over, he looked at me and said, "You definitely have Parkinson's disease." He prescribed some pills for me to take that trick the brain into thinking they are dopamine. He told me that PD is a progressive, degenerative condition which means over time it will continually get worse. The good news he told me was that it isn't fatal. People die with Parkinson's, not from Parkinson's. He also said most people have about 10 years to continue working before the PD symptoms worsen to the point that working is no longer an option. But it's different for everyone. The insidious part is even though it may take 20 years before you know you have it, symptoms start almost immediately after the first cell perishes.

Looking back from here, I recognize what my first symptom was. About 20 years ago I lost my sense of smell. That is a common non-motor symptom of PD. But of course, by itself there is no way to recognize it as a part of Parkinson's. Slowly over the years, more things would show up from time to time that were troubling, but they all seemed unrelated. About 15 years ago, I started really suffering from depression and anxiety for no reason. Life was good. Great wife...great kids...great job...nice house. Life was exceeding my expectations. So why couldn't I enjoy any of it and why was I so miserable. Again, I had no idea depression is a common PD symptom. When people are confronted by something unexplainable and difficult to live with, we develop Coping Mechanisms. They are things we do to make the pain tolerable. Whether the pain comes from physical or mental sickness or heartbreak or loss. Hopefully, the mechanism we develop is a positive one, not alcohol or illegal drugs. For the depression, I developed the habit of walking every day. I found a tree lined road close to my house and I would walk its length and back. Rain or shine, day or night, I would walk. Also, when it was warm out, every Sunday evening I would drive to the prettiest lake and watch the sunset.

I would of course take God with me on these walks and to these sunsets, but He would only listen. I knew He was there and I knew He was hearing me. I trusted Him enough to just let Him stay quiet.

Then one day, my wife and I were walking somewhere. She looked at me and said, " Your left arm isn't swinging when you walk." We walked a little more and sure enough, it wasn't. It just kind of hung there awkwardly. I started to think about all the weird things that had been accumulating over the years and the next time I saw my family doctor, I told him about all of them. When I had finished, he said, " Sounds to me like Parkinson's. That's when he made the appointment for me with the neurologist.

I had two initial reactions to the news that I had PD. First was a profound feeling of relief. What's worse than suffering is suffering for no apparent reason. Now my suffering had a name, Parkinson's disease. Second, I immediately began to develop my coping mechanisms.
It's been a long and ever-changing process. As I lose my ability to do things, I replace them with alternatives when I can. One of the things I

have lost that is the hardest to adjust to is the inability to walk more than a short time. My walk is now a shuffle and after a short time I have to sit. There is also the constant danger of falling, (one of the two main reasons for someone with PD to be hospitalized. The other is choking). So, to keep my spirits up and allow me to get outside and get some exercise, I ride a bike every day. That's my #1 coping

mechanism. Of course, not the two-wheel kind. I would go maybe 2 ft and fall over sideways. Mine has 3 wheels. One in the front and two in the back. It's called a recumbent delta trike.
I thank God for my trike. Other than when I'm sleeping, the only other time I don't feel the Parkinson's is when I'm riding my bike.

P.S. I have discovered that most of the time, God works silently.

I Dream Of Movement

Parkinson's disease is classified as a movement disorder. The human body needs a chemical that certain cells in the brain were designed to produce. That chemical enables the body to move correctly. For some reason, as many as 20 years ago, those cells in my brain started to die. After about 80 percent of them were dead, my body started acting peculiar. It began to ignore what my brain was telling it to do. My body also began doing things my brain was not directing it to do. My body began to rebel. With the demise of those certain brain cells, the authority my brain had over the actions of my body began to break down, but not completely. My brain is still in control for the most part. But slowly, different systems of my body are acting on their own. This is happening with both types of movement, voluntary movement and involuntary movement. With voluntary movement, like walking, my brain tells my legs to move a certain way to achieve a normal walking stride. My legs refuse and start a kind of shuffling movement. Without that chemical those brain cells previously produced, my legs ignore my brain's instructions. They move the way they want too. Then there's involuntary movement, like digestion. When I eat, my brain tells my digestive tract to move the food through my body at a certain rate so the good parts of the food can be used where my body needs it and any waste can be disposed of all in a timely fashion. But again, without that chemical, everything slows down. My brain tells my digestive system to move things along at the normal rate. Instead, the system slows and backs up.

As time goes by, my body's rebellion is intensifying. More systems are affected. My brain's ability to maintain control is being compromised. With others that have this condition, movement has been known to stop. They refer to it as "freezing". A person will be shuffling along and all of a sudden, their legs will just stop. They can't move. When this happens, the persons brain needs a reboot. Many times, this can be accomplished by placing a small obstacle on the floor in front of the frozen person. The presence of this obstacle does something in the person's brain that allows it to direct the legs to move again. Some people with this challenge use a walking cane that will shine a laser beam across their path that appears as an obstacle to the brain and they can move again.

I have heard people say that when an ability is lost, like sight or hearing, the person will dream and in the dreams what they lost is regained. They say the same regarding people that lose a limb. In their dreams, they are whole and can run and throw a ball. When I dream, I dream of movement. My body does what my brain tells it to do when and how my brain tells it to. My body does what my brain tells it to do when and how my brain tells it too.

To get good at any physical activity requires what is called muscle memory. Repeating a certain movement until the body moves that way without even thinking about it. It's necessary to do this if you're learning to shoot a gun well or throw a football. My body has lost its memory. When I dream of movement, I wake and

I remember the feeling of the movement in the dream. Then with the first movement of the day, the truth that my body muscles have lost their memory becomes instantly clear.

They say Parkinson's is not fatal. That's good. I haven't heard of anyone's heart or lungs that have stopped because of the lack of dopamine." That's the name of the chemical that the dead cells produced. So, things could be much worse.

I just have to deal with my dreams keeping the memories of movement alive.

Light Into Darkness

Parkinson's disease is classified as a movement disorder. My brain is lacking the substance that tells my body to move. My body wants to stay still. This gives me a lot more time to sit and think.

I have been thinking about free will lately. I know God gave man a free will. He obviously gave the angels a free will. (Satan used his free will against God and suffered the consequences.) I thought I had come to the conclusion that to have a free will, it was necessary to have the ability to make a wrong choice. Satan and all that followed him made a wrong choice. Adam and Eve made a wrong choice. They chose evil over good.

I thought about heaven. When we get there will we still have a free will, or could it be that we no longer have a free will because heaven is perfect and we will be perfect and not having the option of making a wrong choice.

The only beings with self-awareness I know to exist are God, man and angels. They all have a free will. But if free will requires the option to make a choice between what is right and what is wrong, God would not have a free will because it is impossible for Him to make a wrong choice or to choose evil.

Then I thought about

light and darkness. It is said that darkness is the opposite of light, but it's not. Darkness is the absence of light.

Darkness is not a thing. It is only what happens if you remove light. Evil is not a thing. It is simply what happens when good is removed.

The question is asked, because God created everything, did God create evil? No.

Everything about God and everything from God is good. Evil is the result of removing good. If that is true, then evil is not a choice made by a being with a free will, but the result of a being with a free will doing something that is not good. By their act, they are removed from God and by their act become evil. That is the result of the absence of God. Just like darkness is the result of the absence of light.

I believe that to have a free will is to have the will and freedom to be good, to do good, and the freedom not to do evil and not having to suffer the result of not being good.

As we travel down life's path, from time to time we will come to a fork in the road. We must choose which way to go. Usually the wrong path is smooth and well maintained and heavily travelled. The right path is rough and obviously the path less taken, but we know in our hearts

it's the right way.
Remember, we have the free will to take the right path and the freedom to not take the wrong.
Also remember, those that take the wrong path are not taking it because they have the free will to do it, but because they are struggling in darkness and have been deceived.

The Selfishness Of Sickness

When you have a progressive, degenerative sickness like Parkinson's disease or any long-term health condition or injury, there is a tendency to become selfish. We are told by God to consider other people's needs above our own. Most of my life I have known this command and have tried to live it. Now that I'm sick, I'm finding it more difficult to do. The requirements and demands of the disease are getting in the way. Growing up a Christian trying to live an unselfish life, I know how hard it can be to deny ourselves and put someone else first. I understand why God asked us to do this. It's one of those things that makes sense after the fact. The root of selfishness is pride. Selfishness is loving ourselves instead of loving God and others. When I wasn't sick, being unselfish was something I could choose to be. It was just a matter of making the right choice. There were no obstacles keeping me from choosing to be unselfish. Now, Parkinson's disease is conspiring with my body and brain to look inward rather than outward. Outward to the needs of others is where my gaze should be fixed.

Before my sickness, the moment by moment decisions and needs were mostly under my control. A situation would arise and I was free to decide what to do. A need would present itself, either for me or someone else, and I was free to fulfill or deny the need. What I found out about God was if I kept my attention on the needs of others, my needs would be taken care of. I had very little reason to look inward at my own needs. God always provided. I was free to consider other's needs and the needs of my wife, my children, family, friend's, employers, co-workers and strangers, anyone that crossed my path. Many times, I failed in my attempt to live an unselfish life, but to live unselfishly was my desire.

Today, as I write this I find I am becoming a selfish person. A person that is more and more considering my needs more than the needs of others. I still know that God requires me to consider others more than I consider myself. It's getting harder. When every part of my body is screaming, " I'm in pain," or " I don't want to move," or " I'm going to move whether you want me to or not," it's hard not to fix my gaze inward. When I refer to the selfishness of sickness, I can only speak of Parkinson's disease/ Arthritis. (I have not spoken with many other sick people about what is being screamed at them, but I would imagine the screams are similar to mine and they are also being drawn inward).

These are a few of the obstacles Parkinson's has placed in my path to being unselfish.

Making it difficult to find a place to be comfortable and remain comfortable for more than a short time.

Taking away my ability

to walk more than a few steps without becoming exhausted.

Taking away my ability to stand unaided for more than a few minutes without having to sit.

Taking away my ability to speak loudly and clearly enough for people to understand what I am trying to say. With that, taking away my desire to speak because of frustration and embarrassment.

Taking away my desire for normal conversation because of fatigue and frustration.

Taking away the pleasure of eating out in public because of the fear of choking.

Taking away the pleasure of just leaving my house because of the fear of falling or just getting into a situation out of my control.

These obstacles and others that just show up regularly are making it hard to not be selfish. They cause me to want to always control my surroundings to meet my needs.

I know that God still wants me to do what He has asked us to do. He wants me to love Him. He wants me to trust Him. He wants me to love those around me. Because I am sick, those around me are fewer than before. My ability and opportunity to touch people's lives is diminishing. I also know that being sick does not excuse me from being unselfish.

I was talking with my wife last night. I told her that I was concerned about the future and that my life was getting smaller and smaller and could soon disappear. Her response resulted in one of those moments that had the possibility of changing the course of the rest of my life. She told me I was fortunate and in a unique place. She said most Christians desire to know God better but the tyranny of the immediate, the demands of life and of time does not allow them to spend the time with God that they would like. She said I have been set free from that. Even though my body is bound, my mind and spirit are free to pursue God without limitation.

Now that's interesting. As long as my mind and spirit are free, I am free to live an unselfish life. It doesn't matter if it comes to the point that my body can't leave the house. I can still live the life God wants me to live. I can commit acts of unselfishness despite any obstacle placed in my path.

As I live out the rest of this blink of an eye that's my life here on earth, I will probably be a tad selfish regarding what I must do to live a life with Parkinson's. I may need to use tools to cope with the effects of the disease that will appear to be selfish. But my heart's desire and my resolve will be to consider you and your needs above my own, whenever and however I can.

Healing In A Fallen World

Now some random thoughts on healing. I think I've been sick the normal amount of times over the years I have lived on this earth. That is, normal for someone living in America in the 20th and 21st centurys. I have had many colds, flu, fevers, sore throats, ear aches. I have been in the hospital 4 times... hepatitis, 2 hernias and 1 chest pain, (I think it was heart burn). It doesn't feel good to be sick. When we are sick, we

can't wait to feel good again. And fortunately, after a while, we do. If we injure something or something happens like a hernia or appendicitis, we go to a doctor and get it fixed. But some things aren't fixable and won't go away over time. Cancer, MS, and many other diseases don't usually go away.
I have Parkinson's Disease. They call it a progressive degenerative disease. That means it keeps

getting worse over time and doesn't stop getting worse. They say people don't die from Parkinson's. They die "with" Parkinson's. Something else is the cause of their death.

I believe that God has the ability to supernaturally heal the human body. I believe it has happened many times over history. In the Christian circles I have traveled in all my life, the consensus is that God heals.

But my life experience

shows me that healing is not that easy to get a hold of.

I have thought about this a great deal throughout my life, especially when I'm sick or someone I love is sick. But with the normal everyday sick, even though you are asking God to heal you, in the back of your mind you know that after a while, the sickness will run its course, and you will be well again.

It's not the same with something like

Parkinson's Disease. This doesn't go away. There are things they can do to help make the journey a little easier and hold off the degenerative part for a while, but you can only imagine what's coming. Michael J. Fox says, " Having Parkinson's Disease is like getting hit by a bus, only in slow motion. You see it hitting you, but you can't get out of the way".

Healing takes on a different meaning when

you have something that won't, in the natural, go away. But don't I believe in the supernatural? Don't I believe God has the ability to heal Parkinson's? Of course, He does. He can do anything, can't He? Let's see. Can God lie? No. Can He violate His word? No. Can He be unjust? No. When mankind fell in the garden, we let in everything that can hurt us and cause us sorrow and steal what belongs to us. God gave mankind the world and mankind gave it away and gave the adversary the right to be here and cause us pain and death. One of the things mankind allowed to enter the earth was sickness, disease and injury. We also caused a void to be placed between us and God.

But God loved us so much that He gave His Son to take our place and remove the void that separated us. His Son came to earth and brought with Him restoration and freedom from death. God certified Jesus as His Son by healing people Jesus and those with Him laid their hands on.

In the bible, there are random healings in the Old Testament. There are many healings described in the Gospel's in the New Testament and some random healings in the rest of the New Testament. From the New Testament writers until now, healings have become less understood and experienced. There are many reasons given for the unpredictability of healing, from not having enough faith to receive healing, to the person that is praying for the person in need of healing not having enough faith, or from not praying long enough to not praying hard enough. Some say healing doesn't happen because the sick person will learn a great lesson through having and enduring the sickness and pain, maybe patience or empathy. It's also said that the healing has happened, just hasn't manifested yet.

I have prayed for healing from Parkinson's. I have been prayed for. As of this writing, I still feel the symptoms. If I skip the medication, it gets worse. I love God and Jesus is my savior. I have sinned and will sin again. I don't want to, but I probably will. I could pray more for healing

and be prayed for by others more. I could have more faith, I guess. I'm a little confused where enough is.
I love God, I trust God. I'm doing the best I can to be a good son. I have always felt His love for me. Most of the time, I feel I please Him. I don't think He's mad at me or withholding healing from me. I don't think he is disappointed that I'm not healed. I think I live in a world He made perfect and my first

parents ruined. Even though I'm not subject to death anymore and I will live in perfection with Him forever, for a short time, I will have Parkinson's. But His love for me never fails.

Right Choices Are Hard

I chose to be a follower of Jesus at the age of 6. I know it may be hard to believe that at 6, someone can make that kind of choice. I think it may be my first memory. Someone asked me the question," Do you accept God's sacrifice of His Son for the restoration of the relationship between God and mankind that was lost at the fall of Adam and Eve? Do you repent of all your sins and promise to live the rest of your life for Him and for others? (Wait, I was six! Not much time to sin yet.) I think different words were used. They were along the lines of, " Do you invite Jesus into your heart?" I remember saying yes, and then repeating a simple prayer and finally hearing someone say, "Now you are saved." Ever since that moment, I have lived my life seeing the world through the eyes of a follower of Jesus...my joys, my sorrows, my achievements, my failures, my pain, my pleasure, my sin, my undeserved favor. Every minute of my life has been seen through Christian eyes.

During my years as a Jesus follower, I have learned how to live that life from many different sources, a number of churches I have attended, each having a different flavor than the others. The common denominator is they were all "protestant". The different flavors came from their denominational history, their past and present leadership and how they interpreted what God wanted to say in the bible. I learned from my family, my friends, the books I read and, of course, the Holy Spirit. Over the years, my mind was developed and molded and changed by

all these ingredients.
And now, here I am. With a mind filled with teachings and experiences that I use to interpret my daily life. I have tried to make good decisions each day. Some days I have been more successful at it than other days.
I have determined that for the most part, wherever we are in our lives, most of us are there because of the choices we have made all along the way, good

choices and bad choices. From "Should I go to college," to, "Should I forgive the person who has wronged me ". There is a scene in a movie I like. An older man that has lived a life he is not proud of is talking to a large group of teenagers. He tells them, "As I lived my life, I always knew what the right path was. Without exception, I knew. But I never took it. Do you know why? Because it was too hard." I have found the right choice is usually the hard choice. Doing something you know is right but has a cost. Walking away from something you really want but you know is wrong. Doing something that will diminish you for the benefit of someone that doesn't deserve it. I hope I will always be willing to make the right choices, hard or easy. Whenever confronted by a hard choice, I try to think about how this choice will affect me and those around me, now and in the future. And I remember, God is watching.

Different Universes

Living life in this material world, it is easy to think that all that is real can be experienced through our 5 senses. We think we know what we know by what we see, hear, smell, feel and taste. But there is so much more that is going on beyond the reach of our senses.

We have a body that senses things. We also have a mind that interprets what the body experiences. Another word that describes the mind is soul.

soul
sōl/
noun
noun: soul; plural noun: souls

The spiritual or immaterial part of a human being, regarded as immortal.
a person's moral or emotional nature or sense of identity.
"in the depths of her soul, she knew he would

betray her."
The soul is said to consist of our mind, will and emotions.

We also are a spirit. This spirit is our true selves. When I think, dream, plan, show kindness, act unkind, pray, love, hate...... These are all acts of my spirit.

These three things put together make up who we are. It's like the body is the vehicle we use to act and function in this world. The soul is the power that drives the body and steers it into action based on the information the 5 senses provide. Our spirit is the truest part of us that makes the body and soul do what they do in the context of what we are and know to be true. The soul and spirit are the only two parts of us that are immortal. The body wears out and when it does, we discard it like an old suit.

If we are awake, we are aware of other universe's besides our own. These universes are inhabited by beings that are different than us. They have been around a lot longer than us. In these universes reside angels and demons. They have the ability to move between our universe and theirs. They have the ability to act and influence us and our universe. And they are at war. The war is for our spirits. Most of us are not aware that this war is taking place, even though it has been going on since the garden of Eden.

The war is between good and evil and the prize is us. The war was started by our choosing evil over good, Satan over God.

Fortunately, God loves us so much that despite the fact that we betrayed Him, He is willing to fight to get us back.

The wonderful truth is, He has already won that war. Unfortunately, mankind and Satan don't seem to realize it. Satan and his army continue to try to convince us that the war is still raging. He is still doing everything he can to convince us that he still has power. Any power he has is temporary and actually an illusion. He and his minions continue to fight to convince us to choose his universe over God. But just like our universe, Satan's universe will end. It is already happening.

But the skirmishes continue.

One of my favorite books was written by Frank Peretti. Its title is, "This Present Darkness." Early in the book there's an incident where a small-town Pastor is in his small church praying for his people and his town. It's night. Outside, something is trying to break into the church to get to him. But this something is being closely watched. This is a fictional glimpse into the war that is still being fought over us.

Here is the passage from the book;

The night scene of the quiet street was a collage of stark blue moonlight and bottomless shadows. But one shadow did not stir with the wind as did the tree shadows, and neither did it stand still as did the building shadows. It crawled, quivered, moved along the street toward the church, while any light it crossed seemed to sink into its blackness, as if it were a breach torn in space. But this shadow had a shape, an animated, creature-like shape, and as it neared the church sounds could be heard: the scratching of claws along the ground, the faint rustling of breeze-blown, membranous wings wafting just above the creature's shoulders.

It had arms and it had legs, but it seemed to move without them, crossing the street and mounting the front steps of the church. Its leering, bulbous eyes reflected the stark blue light of the full moon with their own jaundiced glow. The gnarled head protruded from hunched shoulders, and wisps of rancid red breath seethed in labored hisses through rows of jagged fangs. It either laughed or it coughed—the wheezes puffing out from deep within its throat could have been either. From its crawling posture, it reared up on its legs and looked about the quiet neighborhood, the black, leathery jowls pulling back into a hideous death-mask grin. It moved toward the front door. The black hand passed through the door like a spear through liquid; the body hobbled forward and penetrated the door, but only halfway.

Suddenly, as if colliding with a speeding wall, the creature was knocked backward and into a raging tumble down the steps, the glowing red breath tracing a corkscrew trail through the air.

With an eerie cry of rage and indignation, it gathered itself up off the sidewalk and stared at the strange door that would not let it pass through. Then the membranes on its back began to billow, enfolding great bodies of air, and it flew with a roar headlong at the door, through the door, into the foyer—and into a cloud of white hot light. The creature screamed and covered its eyes, then felt itself being grabbed by a huge, powerful vise of a hand. In an instant, it was hurling through space like a rag doll, outside again, forcefully ousted. The wings hummed in a blur as it banked sharply in a flying turn and headed for the door again, red vapors chugging in dashes and streaks from its nostrils, its talons bared and poised for attack, a ghostly siren of a scream rising in its throat. Like an arrow through a target, like a bullet through a board, it streaked through the door— And instantly felt its insides tearing loose. There was an explosion of suffocating vapor, one final scream, and the flailing of withering arms and legs. Then there was nothing at all except the ebbing stench of sulfur and the two strangers, suddenly inside the church.

The big blond man replaced a shining sword as the white light that surrounded him faded away.

More Like Jesus

I have a personality trait that has driven my wife crazy ever since we first met. Sometimes I tend to be a tad secretive. I either keep information from her or I give her only partial information. I will also say things for effect. I don't think I do this maliciously, though I would have a hard time convincing her of that.

Sometimes I will not inform her about a purchase I have made. I think I do that because I don't want to make my case for the reason for the purchase. I know I will get some resistance from her. A lot of the time I will return that item and she never knows the transaction occurred. If I do decide to keep it, I would rather make my case after the fact.

Other times I will leave out or not mention information regarding events in our lives. They may or may not affect her directly or indirectly.

I really don't know why I do this. It may be an attempt to control some part of our lives. It could be something I know she will react to adversely. I always try to avoid being in the path of that!

I do know I would never withhold anything that she needs to know.... Something that would endanger or hurt us. I do try to avoid this trait but it does still happen from time to time.

I will also say things just to get a rise out of her. Sometimes I enjoy her reaction, sometimes it backfires.

We were talking this morning about Jesus and I had a thought. Jesus also had this trait.
Not the purchasing part, but the giving limited information part and saying things for effect. I told Marcia that I was just trying to be more

like Jesus!

As I think about the life of Jesus, there does seem to be times when he would leave people guessing, and also say something for effect.

It's like the parables. Many times, as I read them I think, why doesn't He just say what He means. His disciples always seemed to be wondering about what he was saying and doing.

He told a woman with a sick child that He was not there for her and basically called her a dog. I don't really think that's what He thought. He was looking for a reaction. She reacted rightly.

Then there is the time He told Peter he was the rock that the church would be built upon. A verse or two later He called Peter Satan and to get out of His way. I don't think Jesus thought

Peter was Satan. He said it for affect. When Jesus gathered his men for their last meal before He was to be killed, he told them they must eat His body and drink His blood. They wondered what in the world did that mean?

After He had risen, the disciples were left wondering what had happened. They and others had seen Jesus, but He would just pop in and out. Peter decides, "

I'm going fishing." After fishing all night, they caught nothing. As the sun was coming up, a man on the shore yells to them, " How's the fishing?" They answered, " No good." The man on the shore told them to cast their net on the right side of the boat this time.

They pulled the net in full of fish. They realized it was Jesus. They cooked breakfast and ate together. Jesus took Peter aside to talk. During the conversation Jesus told Peter how he would die. Peter noticed John and asked Jesus, "How will he die?" Jesus responded, " If I want him to live until I return, what business is that to you?" That started the rumor that John would never die.

We are told to be like Jesus. He did seem to say and do things for effect. I'm really not saying what I do because of this trait in me is an effort on my part to be like Jesus.

What I am saying is that my desire is to be like Jesus, in love, compassion, mercy and all the positive traits that He wants to see in my life.

Microscopic Adversaries

I have always known that this body and this mind were fragile. As with most people, my body gets sick. Some microscopic result of the fall of man invades my system from time to time and I get sick.

Thankfully, God provided an additional provision for this. I guess I would call it an after the fall gift. Before the fall, Adam and Eve did not have an immune system. They didn't need one. They were perfect and there were no germs. After the fall, their bodies needed something to fight off these invaders of the fall, so they were provided with body defenses to battle these new enemies. It's been war ever since. These germs and bacteria attacking and adapting. Our defenses fighting back and adapting. Throughout history, our microscopic foes have tried many times to wipe us out. So far, our immune systems and the intelligence God has given to man to invent defenses have kept us from obliteration. I'm frankly surprised we are still here. If Satan had his way, we wouldn't be.

When I was younger, despite getting sick, I did have a feeling of invincibility. That ended for me at the age of 50. That's the year I believe I started to feel the presence of Parkinson's disease. Any feeling of invincibility ended. My body and my mind were telling me something was wrong. More wrong than anything I had previously felt. Not knowing what was wrong was the worst part. It played havoc with my brain, body and my mind. I not only suffered from the onslaught of my physical body and brain being attacked by this unknown assailant, but my mind was fighting depression. Only after the adversary had been identified did a strange peace and resolve descend upon me. I was not imagining the things that were happening to me and the depression is a symptom of Parkinson's.

So, roughly 15 years ago, for some reason unknown to me, my brain started to cut back its production of dopamine. That's the chemical the brain produces to aid and regulate movement. As the production decreases, my body moves slower. And not only my body and muscles, but some of my internal systems also. Digestion is one example. The little flap that insures what's supposed to go to the stomach goes to the stomach, and what's supposed to go to the lungs goes to the lungs, is another. It gets slow and I tend to choke. They say that by the time a person starts to notice any Parkinson's symptoms, about 80% of their dopamine producing brain cells are dead.

My journey with Parkinson's disease started with symptoms from an unknown cause when I was 50, diagnosed when I was 54. But the journey hasn't been too bad so far. Yes, I have had to stop working, I now drive very rarely. I'm slow, I'm tired all the time and get exhausted easily. Each day I become less dependent on what I have always been able to do and more dependent on my wife Marcia to stand in for me in life. But that's ok. I could spend my time mourning the loss of me and feeling guilty for having to add all these things to Marcia's plate. The bottom line though is that I didn't ask for this. It just turned out to be my journey. And my sweet wife is just that, my sweet wife. She chose to walk this life with me. I would do the same for her.

My immune system can't fight this. There are a lot of smart people working on a cure for Parkinson's. If that proves to be too elusive, they are also working on finding a way to prevent it and tools to help people like me live our lives to the fullest.

As I continue to travel down this road that God did not want me to travel down, but was created by rebellion against God, I can see the white shores of my destination. It is more beautiful than words can describe. If I look real hard, I think I can see a crowd standing on the shore, waving me on.

And I do know that as my feet touch that sand and I go to greet all those I love, I will be running!

Naked

This morning while I was in the shower, I started to think about being naked. The state of being naked is one area that, more than most areas of our lives, is a reality that shows the creativity of God and the wickedness of the devil.

Nakedness has more facets than a gemstone. Its effect touches so many areas of the human experience.

All of us are born naked. We come into this world unadorned and uncovered and, of course, unaware that we are. When God made the first man, the man started the same way, naked and unaware. Adam and Eve ran around the garden unconcerned that they were naked. As Adam and God walked and talked in the cool of the day, Adam was naked. I'm not sure if God wore anything, but we know Adam didn't think twice about being clothing free.

Then the devil interfered. He convinced Adam and Eve that God was holding back something good from them. God had told them not to do something, but the devil said it was ok to disobey God.

That evening when God went to meet Adam for their walk, Adam was nowhere to be found. God found him hiding in the bushes. When God asked him why he was hiding, he told God it was because he was naked.

I'm not sure why Adam and Eve's disobedience resulted in the awareness that they were naked. It just tells us they started wearing clothes. I don't think Adam and Eve minded seeing each other naked. I guess they just didn't want God or the animals to see them naked.

Since Adam and Eve, being naked has had a profound effect on human history, good and bad.

Most of the pivotal events in the world's history has involved nakedness.

Again, we are all born naked. As soon as we enter the world, somebody puts something on us. Not so much to cover up the cute little parts of a naked baby, but to keep us warm. From then on, we spend most of our time with some kind of covering. To protect us from the elements and to cover parts of us that most of us don't want other people to see. Depending on our age in life, there are exceptions.

When we are a baby, like Adam and Eve before the fall, we are unaware of our nakedness. Our moms and dads and caregivers do have an awareness of nakedness, but out of relationship and necessity, our nakedness is natural. As we get older and become self-aware, our awareness of our own nakedness is apparent. Most of us don't want others to see us naked.

Now for this next part, there are two basic elements. Nakedness the way God intended and nakedness perverted by mankind and the devil. Being a man, of course this will be from a male's perspective.

One day, usually during the early teen years, boys make the discovery that they are drawn to a desire to see a naked girl. This desire is both mental and physical. And it is strong. And it is part of God's plan. Unfortunately, most boys are unprepared for this tsunami of thoughts and feelings. Being unprepared and lacking the wisdom of knowledge that every boy should have been given, they get swept away in this wave of desire. They only know that their body and brain are screaming, " Naked is good!" They are unaware that God has provided boundaries of protection where they can be safe. They are also unaware that the devil knows every man's weakness and has invested unimaginable resources and personnel to make sure men are destroyed by something God created for good.

So rather than a boy growing up to be a man that is able to find the right woman for him, both protected and intact so they can enjoy a healthy and blessed state of nakedness together, the boy gets swept up in the unnatural pursuit of nakedness that can destroy his life and future.

As we start to walk down the path of life towards our sunset, it's as though we go back in time to childhood. Our awareness of nakedness becomes less and less as the days pass by. If we live long enough, we again reach a point where our awareness of our own nakedness ceases to exist. Someone puts something on us for protection and warmth. The difference from a baby is that someone puts something on us to cover the wrinkly parts of our bodies no-one wants to see.

Nakedness, ours or anyone else's no longer matters.

In A Heartbeat

For reasons unknown to me, God thought a thought. The thought was to make a universe, so large that it has no boundaries. At a location of His choosing, He placed a sphere that would travel in space moving in a cosmic dance in step with the rest of the universe. He made the surface of this sphere according to a plan. He intended to place a being of His creation on the surface of the sphere. The being was designed to live and thrive in this place.

When this universe was prepared and the sphere was in its place and ready, God formed a likeness of Himself on the surface of the sphere out of the same material He used to create the universe. He blew one of His breaths into what He had formed. Something happened that had never happened before. There was a new sound in the universe. It was a new note in this symphony he was creating. It was a beat. It was the first heartbeat. It echoed throughout the universe. This first beat was followed by a second. Then by a third. And so, it began.

Soon after, this heartbeat was joined by another. And then another, until today the universe is filled with the sound of billions of heartbeats.

The sound of a new

heartbeat is the sound of promise. The promise of a new life. If the heartbeat is allowed to continue to beat, the reason the first beat was heard can come into being. If the heartbeat is stopped, all the potential and purpose will be lost. God's purpose for the first beat will be lost.

Every new heartbeat holds the potential for greatness. Each new heartbeat holds the potential for evil. How each heart is cared for by the one who holds the heartbeat within their chests and those around them determines which it will be. If a heartbeat is protected and loved, the possibilities for good are unlimited. A heartbeat that is not protected is always in danger both for the one who's chest holds the heartbeat and those around.

Just as every new heartbeat beats with the rhythm of promise and echoes through the universe, every heartbeat that stops means the end. The end of a life lived in harmony with other heartbeats or the end of a life lived out of rhythm. A heartbeat in harmony creates beauty and life. A heartbeat lived out of rhythm creates chaos, destruction and even the silencing of heartbeats.

Long ago, God gave something of Himself to a young woman. Not long after, another new heartbeat was heard. This one sounded different. This one had the potential for good and the promise of freedom for all heartbeats that chose to beat in harmony with it. This so threatened hearts that beat out of rhythm that they conspired together to stop this heartbeat. They succeeded in their intent to stop this heart from beating. They went so far as to thrust the point of a spear into this heart to make sure it would never beat again. They placed this silenced heart into a stone cave and sealed the entrance with a large round stone.

Three days later a sound could be heard coming from inside the cave. It was a heartbeat. They rolled the stone back and found the cave was empty.
The sound of this heartbeat signaled freedom from death for

everyone that believed the heartbeat was true.

When a life ends, a heartbeat stops. The universe becomes a little quieter. Those hearts that choose to beat in harmony with the heartbeat that escaped the cave go on forever. Those that choose to beat out of rhythm and harmony will be lost.

Guard your heart so it will beat in time with the symphony of God.

We Serve At The Pleasure Of The King

It is spring. "The season when kings go off to war." Our king has sent us to capture a city and destroy a people. In this season, our king is not with us. He has chosen to remain in his palace and send us, his army, to fight without him. We serve at the pleasure of the king.

I serve under a commander I greatly respect. He has led us to victory so many times. When I was young and joined the king's army, my father had recently died and the commander became much more than a commander to me. I look up to him as a father and he considers me his son.

Three days ago, my commander said He had a message from the King. To my surprise, he told me the message was for me. He said that the King had summoned me and I was ordered to go to the king's palace immediately. I gathered a few things and started to run. It was a day's journey by foot to the palace. I arrived late in the evening. I approached the entrance to the palace and told the guard who I was and that the King had summoned me. He instructed two of his fellow guards to escort me to the king. They led me to a large room. They announced me. From behind a curtain appeared the king. All of us bowed and the King dismissed my escort. The king walked across the room and sat on a finely made sofa and motioned for me to sit beside him. He was a very impressive looking man, made more impressive by what I had witnessed him do in battle and the many stories I had heard regarding the many brave and heroic feats he had performed over the years. I sat and looked at his face, but respectfully, I did not look directly into his eyes.

He asked me questions regarding how the war was going and how the men were doing. Then he said, " I have a task for you, but it's late and I'm tired. Go home tonight, get cleaned up and I will send for you in the morning". Then he rose from the sofa, turned and left the room. Right after he left, the two guards that had escorted me earlier came in and escorted me out of the palace. When I got outside, I was about to start walking towards home when a thought came into my mind. I can't go home. My commander and the army were out on the battle field. How could I go home and sleep comfortably knowing they were out there? I turned around and walked back to the entrance of the palace and asked one of the guards that was warming himself by a fire if it would be all right if I found a corner out of the way and rolled my mat out to spend the night. After giving me a puzzled look he gave me his permission. So, I spent the night among the king's servants.

When morning came. I got up, rolled up my sleeping mat and looked around thinking about what I should do next. I saw one of my escorts from yesterday across the courtyard and walked over to him.

When he saw me approaching, he turned to me and asked, "Where have you been? We went to your house this morning to bring you to the King. Your wife told us she hadn't seen you and thought you were still with the army." I told him I had slept here last night. After another puzzled look, he again escorted me to the King.

When we arrived at the room, he left me at the

door and walked to the other side of the room where the King was standing. They spoke to each other for a short time and then the guard left the room. The king pointed to the same sofa we had sat on yesterday and we both sat down. He asked me, where did you spend the night last night. I told him I slept in the entrance of the palace. He asked me why I would sleep there rather than go to my house to sleep. I told him the reason and he gave a quiet chuckle. Then he said to me, " Don't be concerned about that. No one would consider you spending a night at home with your family a betrayal to your comrades in the field. Tomorrow you will leave for the camp. I will have something for you to deliver to the commander. In the meantime, I am gathering with a few men on my staff tonight. I would like you to be there. Come back at sunset. Again, he left the room and my escorts came to show me out.

I spent the day at the market and with a longtime friend. He was surprised when he saw me, knowing I was away with the army. We speculated as to why the King had summoned me but came up with nothing.

Just before sunset, I returned to the palace

and joined the gathering of men, trying to make conversation but finding it difficult. I felt out of place. For some reason, I started to feel like the goose that had been invited to dinner.

From the time I arrived, the servants started serving many different types of wine. All evening there were toasts to everything imaginable. The king seemed very insistent that I keep my glass empty so the servants could continuously fill it. It wasn't very long before I discovered I was getting very drunk. When the evening came to an end, I think I remember my escorts having to carry me out of the palace.

I awoke in the middle of the night and found myself lying on the stoop in front of my house. I remembered what the King had said earlier in the day about not feeling

I was betraying my friends, but I couldn't get past the thought in my heart that I was. So, I turned from the front door of my house and slowly made my way back to the entrance of the palace. There I found my sleeping mat where I had left it, rolled it out and went to sleep.

The next thing I remember is someone shaking me and talking very loud. My head was pounding and I had a hard time opening my eyes. When I did get them to open, the face of one of my escorts slowly came into focus. He was telling me to get up. I slowly got up and gathered my things. The guard watched me as I put myself together. In his hand was a sealed couriers bag. He handed it to me and instructed me to deliver the bag directly to my commander. He told me that this order came from the King and time was of the essence.

Without hesitation, I started to run. I knew I could make it back to our camp before dark. The day went by without incident.

When I arrived at our camp I went straight to the commander's tent. I announced my presence and he invited me in. He was standing over a table reviewing a map with three of his officers. He welcomed me back and offered me his hand in greeting. I acknowledged the other men and handed the bag to the commander. He took it from me and then returned his attention to the map. I quietly turned and left.

That night as I tried to sleep, my mind kept replaying the last few days trying to figure out what had happened and why the King had summoned me.

The next morning, the army prepared for the days battle. When we were ready, the commander stepped forward and announced that I would be given the honor of leading the charge. As we formed our ranks, I took the forward position. This must have been the message that I had delivered from the King. But why was I awarded this honor? I looked to see if I could find my commander. When I found him, he was looking straight at me. I was taken back by the look on his face. This man I love as a father had the shadow of fear on his face and what appeared to be tears in his eyes.

We heard the blast of the enemy's battle call. We took our positions and started to advance towards the opposing army. I could see the force that was coming towards us was formidable. When the call to charge was given, I pressed forward and felt confident because of the honor given to me by the King and the commander.

Just before we were about to engage the enemy, I gazed to each side of me and then behind me to draw strength from my fellow warriors. But instead of drawing strength, I felt hopelessness and despair. For at that moment I discovered that I was completely alone. My commander and my fellow warriors had turned back and abandoned me to face the enemy alone. Almost immediately I felt the pain of two arrows piercing into my chest. I stumbled and fell to my knees.

I can feel the warmth of the sun on my face and I see it's brilliant light shining off the sword that is whistling through the air on its straight and true path to cut off my head.

I believe these are the last words I will utter in this world,

" I serve at the pleasure of the King!"

Re: 2 Samuel 11 (Bible)

Words

The first time I <u>really</u> heard the words Parkinson's Disease, they were being used by my doctor to describe something that was happening inside me, inside my skin. He spoke the words in response to my description of some unusual challenges I had been facing. I guess I would call them symptoms. Things like my left arm didn't swing when I walked. I had lost my sense of smell. I felt a slight tremor in my left hand. He spoke the words to me in a sentence, "It sounds like you may have Parkinson's disease." It's one of those moments that comes along once in a while that changes the entire direction of our lives, though I didn't realize it at the time.

Normally life happens predictably. I grew up trying to make choices I hoped would result in a good and happy life. I went to school. I tried to do well. I tried to figure out what I wanted to do to make a living. I searched for someone I could love. Because of my parents, my church and my relationship with God and by just paying attention, I discovered early that good made more sense than bad. Bad may have pleasure, but the result of being bad would eventually be bad. Doing good just seemed like the intelligent way to live. It's not that I always made the right choice and never did bad things. It almost always proved that doing bad things resulted in more bad things happening. Doing what I believed to be the right thing resulted in my life being better, both for me and the people my life touched. It just didn't make sense to me to do bad things.

I did discover that making good choices didn't mean that bad things wouldn't still happen to me. Like most people, I wanted to be happy and successful. Happiness is different for everyone. I found out that what makes me happy can be different than what makes someone else happy. What success looks like is different for everyone. As I live my life I make moment to moment decisions that will determine my own happiness and success.

But then come the

moments that will try to destroy the happy and successful life I have been living and pursuing. Usually these moments arrive with words, words spoken by me or spoken to me by others. Words spoken by me like, "Yes, I will do that," to something I know is wrong. "No, I won't do that", to something I know is right. These moments change not only the course of my life, but also change me forever.

Words that are spoken by others, both good and bad, can also change my life and me forever. Like the words, "I don't love you and I don't want to be married to you anymore." Those words were so powerful that from the moment they hit the air, their impact changed the course of my life immeasurably. Those words and the actions and choices that led up to them being uttered caused the life I had planned on to cease to exist, leaving me barely able to stand, staring at a blank canvas.

When I regained my balance, someone else spoke a word to me that again altered the course of my life in ways I could never have imagined. Only this time the word was good. The word was spoken in response to a question I had just asked. The question was, "Will you marry me?" She answered my question with one word, "Yes." The moment that one word hit the air, its impact changed the course of my life immeasurably.

I had heard the words "Parkinson's disease" before. I had heard that some celebrities said they have it. I remembered watching a movie titled "Awakenings" that was about people with Parkinson's. Until those words were spoken to me about me, they were only words. I basically knew what they meant, but they were only words like so many other words. Words that existed to describe something that really didn't affect my life. Now these two words that I had barely thought about were elevated to the status of being two of the primary words used to define me. And as time goes by, how they affect me grows stronger.

I am at a point in my life that my Parkinson's body and brain are steering me down a path that has been travelled by many people before me, but it's all new to me. And like most of life, the ability of others that have traveled this path to be a guide to me is limited. Parkinson's attacks each person in many different ways. The people in my life, my family and friends can encourage me as I walk this path. Without God and Marcia, it would be impossible to go down this road. God is the foundation on which I have tried to build my life and He provides the strength to face everything. Marcia is the love of my life. From the moment she said yes, my life has risen far above my expectations, despite the challenges of living in this fallen world.

On the day Marcia and I were married, we said

words to each other. Living in a "modern world", we decided not to use the traditional vows but instead wrote our own words to say to each other. The words were spoken as a promise. Words that were spoken out loud and witnessed by our family and friends. Usually, these words are referred to as vows. We were making a vow to act and live a certain way for and with each other. The words were based on our love. Words that up until that moment were only words now had weight and substance and power. Words that would change our lives forever. Words that would result in the creation of new life.

I know when Marcia and I said these words to each other, they changed from words into truth. They came to life.

Unfortunately, we have

forgotten the words. We have lost them. When we moved into our first apartment, Marcia embroidered two wall hangings. One with my words to her, one with her words to me. But over the years, they too have been lost.

What happens when you lose words that changed your life and words that you have built so much upon.

I spoke my words to

Marcia in love and because of love. Also with the desire to make a happy life with her.

I remember what my intention was when I spoke the words to her. I promised to love her forever, with an exclusive love only for her. Rejecting all others. I think I said something about leading and protecting her. Also, something about putting her needs before mine. Even though we don't remember the words, the spirit of the words endure.

A man I have known and respected for over 30 years has a saying, "Words mean things". He usually says it when referring to a question about a contract. I think it's even more true when you are talking about wedding vows. What Marcia and I said to each other were not the words of a contract between two people, we made a covenant with each other.

Most traditional marriage vows have words like, "In sickness and in health, till death do us part." I can't remember if we said that to each other. It has always been my intention that Marcia is going to be stuck with me until one of us dies, even though I don't remember saying words that meant that. When you are young and healthy, you can say words like "till death" and absolutely mean them and not really think about the fact that in the blink of an eye you could be at the edge of that cliff staring into the void.

I don't think I'm standing at the edge yet, but the fog has rolled in. It's beginning to get dark and I can sense the void. Parkinson's disease up to this point has been something in my life that

I have been able to cope with, but as it continues to slowly steal things from me, it is getting harder to see. I have been able up until now to find things to replace what the creep is stealing.

I am having trouble walking and getting out of the house, but I have a Segway that I can use to get out on my own and go almost anywhere. Speaking and listening is becoming harder, but there are things like texting that I can still do. I can no longer work. The strange thing is that as I move slower, the days seem to go faster so it's easier to fill up days so I'm not finding myself getting bored. Driving is becoming a challenge, but I can still drive short distances, and we have a golf cart and my Segway. (I wouldn't be able to write this if it weren't for technology, (iPad, slide typing…).

I'm still able to think fairly well. One of the reasons I'm writing this is because I want to think about some things while my head is still clear.

I'm not so much concerned about what's ahead for me as much as I'm concerned about what's ahead for Marcia.

The last song the singer Glenn Campbell recorded before he was pulled into the oblivion of Alzheimer's is titled, "I'm Not Gonna Miss You."

At the time they recorded the song, I don't think he knew what the words he was singing were saying. Someone had to stand beside him and point the words out as he sang. The writers of the lyrics said they wrote the song knowing what he and others suffering with Alzheimer's and those they loved faced. It's harder on the ones that

love the sick person
because the sick person
is unaware that they
don't remember anyone.
The loved ones do
remember but are not
remembered.
Parkinson's disease can
have dementia as a
symptom. How extreme
or how mild it may affect
me is a mystery.

Now I come back to the
words Marcia and I
spoke to each other. I do
remember offering her
all that I am and all that I

have. I also remember putting her needs before my needs.

The bible says we are to esteem others better than ourselves. Jesus also said, "There is no greater love than to lay down your life for a friend. As Parkinson's takes my life from me, I am keenly aware that it is also taking away Marcia's life from her. I love her so much that I would like to free her from having to give up a life of living the adventure that is available to her. It is going to be hard for me to watch her having to sacrifice her life for me. There is so much more she can do over the next 25 years than caring for me. I don't think the promises we made to each other obligated her to this level of sacrifice.

Because of my love for her, I would like to be able to find a way to free her from this future.
I don't think I have the

option of removing myself from this world. I think the Catholics believe that is a one way express ticket to hell. I'm not quite so sure. I don't believe that someone that throws themselves on to a live grenade to save others from death or injury is condemned for doing that. Isn't not wanting Marcia to be trapped into a full-time caregiver's life at the cost of sacrificing a fulfilling, exciting life full of experiences and friendship and ministry considering her needs over my own? I can't get over the idea of her losing her ability and freedom to live out the potential of her gifts and skills due to the fact that she is encumbered by something she didn't sign up for. I would need to be very selfish to let her do that.

Is there another way to free her? Paying people to care for you is something people do. A man I knew for 30 years developed Parkinson's like symptoms when he was 75 years old. Early on, he voiced concerns about his wife having to deal with this, but his wife died of cancer when he was 80 and was still pretty self-sufficient. After his wife died, his Parkinson's progressed rapidly. At 82 he could no longer walk and was confined to a wheelchair and his bed. He had to move out of his house and lived in an assisted living facility with a 24 hour nurse to care for him until he died at the age of 85. Fortunately for him, he was quite wealthy and had options. Marcia and I don't have the option of being able to afford to pay someone to look after me.

Unless God decides to take me home or they come up with a cure, I can't seem to think of a way for Marcia and me to get out of the way of this bus that is hurtling

at us in slow motion.
If I could, I would proclaim to the whole world my love for my wife. If a way cannot be found to free her from this burden, it will take more than an eternity for me to express my love and gratitude for her sacrifice of her life for mine.

The bible could say, " There is no greater love than for a wife to lay down her life for her husband."

Simply Human

Despite the differences in appearance, hair color…. eye color…. skin color…. male or female, we are all born the same. We are simply human.

Not a part of a group or tribe or color or anything else. Nothing that would distinguish us from any other human that has ever lived or will ever live. Anything that labels us was put there, by ourselves or someone else. The truest connection we all have is that we are all born lost. The only thing that really matters is will we remain lost.

We will all die.

After we are dead, we will all stand before God. Everyone. The place where we will stand will be flat and level. There will be no status or position or labels. We will all be the same.

We will all be asked one question. It will not be

one of these;

What did you eat or what did you refrain from eating?
What did you touch or what did you avoid touching?
What did you do or what didn't you do?
What group were you a part of?

The question that will be asked will be, "Did you believe Jesus?"

If the answer is yes, the reason it's yes will not be because of anything done or not done during our life. Except for one thing. Did we believe Him and what He did?

There is a question that could be asked, but won't be asked. "What evidence can be offered to prove your belief in Jesus?" If the question was asked, the answer would be "None." But the question won't be asked.

Evidence will not be presented. If evidence were to be allowed to be presented, it would not include eating this or not eating that, doing this good thing or doing that bad thing. It could include a life of loving God with everything. A life of loving others more than loving ourselves.

I believe that one of the gifts God gave everyone through Jesus was freedom and simplicity.

In all my years of knowing Jesus, the truth is, for myself and many others I have met along the way, trying to figure out what God wants to say to me, "Me", has been a challenge that kept me in a place of frustration and confusion for a long time.

Then I realized something. God's desire and expectation for everyone is to know Him and His Son. He would not have made it hard to do this. He would not

expect this of us and desire this of us and then hide. He gave us a book that we could hold in our hands and understand. He wanted to tell us where we have been, where we are now and where we are going.
I'm still somewhat puzzled about where we have been and why He did some of the things he did and the way he did them. I'm pretty clear on where we are now and I do know where I'm going.

For the where we came from, I just need to trust Him to help me understand the things that I need to understand.

For the where we are now, I'm thankful to Him for the Holy Spirit that speaks to my spirit the deep mysteries and the simple truths of living a life for God and for other people. And as for knowing where I'm going, I'm thankful to Jesus for providing the way and the assurance of it.

I do understand that God would have wanted us to have made different choices, starting with our first parents saying no to the serpents offer. But they said yes. And even though they said yes, God still loved us. He loved us enough to provide a way for all of us to be able to come to a point in our lives where we have the opportunity to choose Him over something else. The same offer our first parents were given. And we are free to make the choice.

God's plan has always been the same, to win us back. To save us from making the wrong choice. The bible is the story of Him doing that. It is a story with many different parts that take place over thousands of years. Much of the story applies to me directly and much of it applies to me indirectly.

This is what the bible story is;

Once upon a time, God created everything. He created a man and a woman. The man and woman had the ability to make a choice. To choose between God or something else. They chose something else. That choice separated the man and woman from God. The man and woman were now lost. All their children would be born lost. But God wanted them back. So, He made a way back. It would take a long time and the journey would be costly. So costly, that it would mean the death of His Son. But God loved us so much, He was willing to pay the price. God's willingness to do this gave every man the right to make the choice between God and something else. Everyone has the opportunity to make the choice. Hopefully a better choice than our first parents made. During the journey from our first parents until this moment, God has been working at restoring us to Him. He separated groups of people from each other by language and color. He made rules for men to follow for protection and direction until they were no longer needed. He sent his Son to restore us to Himself. He sent us a counselor to show us how to love and live. And he has prepared a perfect place for us to be with Him and each other forever.

What gives us the right to enter this place is not who we are or what we have or haven't done or how much we had or didn't have. The right is a gift freely given simply by loving God and His Son and living a life that shows it, and by loving others more than ourselves and living a life that shows it.

Everyone that tries to add extra requirements

for entry into this perfect place are wasting their time. Everyone that tries to earn the right to enter by what they do or refrain from doing will remain lost forever without God.

That's simply the Bibles story.

So, when God asks us the only question we will be asked to answer, what will our answer be? Remember, it will be a yes or no question.

Words (2)

It's hard to look through the eyes of someone else. Even if that someone is the love of your life that has known you and you have known for over 30 years. It's even harder the think through their brain. You may think you know what they are thinking, but you never know. Because you love them so much and have lived so much life together, you always wonder.

Two people find each

other. They fall in love and they get married. On the wedding day, they make promises to each other. They say to each other that these promises will last as long as they live. After the promises are exchanged, they walk down the aisle and usually go to a large room that has been decorated just for them. They are no longer individuals only. They are also something that is singular in nature. Life begins.

With this basic foundation, their lives are lived. They have some idea how they would like life to go. They make their plan. They soon discover unexpected events change their course. They are forced to go a different way.
Sometimes as they travel down the road they choose to go a different way. Because promises were made and distance has been traveled,

everyone's hope is that whatever comes along to cause a change in direction, they will make those changes together.

There are changes you choose. There are changes that just happen. There are changes you can anticipate and plan for. There are changes you know are coming but choose to ignore until they happen.

For Marcia and me,

Parkinson's disease is a change that just happened. I don't know how we could have anticipated it. I don't know of anything we did to cause it to happen. Because we know we live in a fallen world where people grow old and get sick, we knew there was a good chance that if we lived long enough, something would get one of us. It just happened to be me.

When you are just

starting your married life together, your thoughts and actions are filled with jobs, houses, cars, kids, vacations, paying bills, buying musical instruments, going to church and millions of the little moments that come together to make a life. It's you and your mate, taking on each of those moments as they occur. A partnership. A team.

And then you blink. You open your eyes to find

that all of your kids are married. You have a grandson and another grandson on the way. Your career is over. You and Marcia are living in a senior citizen community. Just the two of you and a dog. And you have Parkinson's. Now this is a big change in direction!

The world has changed its axis. What use to be up is now down. Almost everything you called your life is now different.

The number of things you have been able to do whenever you wanted to do them is getting smaller by the minute. Is that old, shaky man looking back at you in the mirror each morning really you?

But enough about me. How about Marcia! Her world has changed axis also. And I have an idea it's tougher for her. Yes, l feel it in my skin but she has to watch it happen. It must be like watching

your love getting hit by a bus in slow motion. The feeling of helplessness to do anything to prevent it. And at the same time, mourning the loss of a life you were looking forward to.
I'm sure she is anticipating the huge challenges she can only imagine, but already seeing a glimpse.

Promises...spoken and meant when we were so young and looking forward to life. We never knew that these promises were for today. We would actually have to act on them.

My choice would be to release her from those promises, but I need her. I would rather she have the freedom to pursue a life filled with fun and fulfillment. The promise does not allow for that. A side of me wants to go back to that day she made the promise to me and eliminate it from our vows. But another side of me is selfish and glad she is with me on this journey we did not choose.

Parkinson's is like playing chess with an opponent that keeps changing the rules with each movement of the pieces. And you can't learn by watching others around you playing chess because their rules are completely different and also changing. Marcia and I don't know how I will act as the result of Parkinson's. I can't warn her that something weird is going to happen because I don't know that it is. Plus, Marcia has always said she never knows what I will do. She has a hard time figuring out what's Parkinson's and what's just me being me. I tend to do things she doesn't understand and I have a difficult time trying to explain myself. One day my memory is ok and the next I can't remember if I took my pills 5 minutes ago. One day I'm an amusing, entertaining person that's fun to be around. The next, sensitive, cranky, chip on my shoulder looking for a fight.

Unfortunately, as I grew older, Marcia also grew older. I'm a older person with Parkinson's along with the physical challenges of being older. Marcia is a very attractive older person with less strength and stamina than someone younger, which is normal. But she not only has to deal with the normal challenges of an older person's life, now add the increased load of making up for my inability to physically work around the house. She also is increasingly having to help me do the simple tasks of life. Taking care of myself. And that will only get worse.

Here we are, two people that love each other

deeply. My love for her wishing I had never put her in this situation, wanting somehow to relieve her of this burden. Her love for me, willing to make a promise all those years ago and now choosing to keep it.

Marcia,

I honor you and I thank you with all my heart for the life of joy you have given to me, for your willingness to walk the rest of this journey with me, though you may have to carry me much of the way.

Just Out Of Reach

Parkinson's disease is referred to as a movement disorder.

The term movement disorder to me means that the human body is unable to move normally. Due to damage of certain cells in the brain, the brain - body connection is broken. The brain continues to send signals to the body to move, but the path these signals must travel is compromised.
This affects my life in a

number of ways.
I am no longer able to sleep with my wife in our bed. Because of pain, I have found the only place I can get a good night sleep and not wake up in the morning in extreme pain is to sleep in a recliner. I first started to discover the various aspects of having a movement disorder from that chair.
When every movement you make is uncomfortable in some way, you find yourself

making less and less movements. My recliner has become a kind of refuge. I have placed it in the middle of the room and I have tried to place all the things around me that I need to have close... IPad, phone, pills, water, remotes for my different devices, my pillows and blankets, paper towels and so on. Because there are so many things I need around me, and just so much space, I try to place everything carefully. But still, I continually find that something I need is just out of my reach. It's frustrating. This morning I reached for a pillow that had fallen on the floor. I tried to reach over from my chair and get it, but it was just an inch too far away. No matter how much I stretched, I couldn't reach it. I had to get up out of the chair, get it and then sit back down again. But, I had my pillow, my blanket and my iPad on my lap. So, it was necessary to lift these things off my lap, find a close place to set them so I could easily reach them when I returned. Painfully and slowly I pushed the lever to lift myself into a sitting position in my recliner. Painfully and slowly tried to stand up, making it on my third attempt. I retrieved the pillow and reversed the painful process to return to my original position in my chair. I was now exhausted, hoping I

hadn't forgotten something.
I'm not lazy. When every movement you make meets with resistance and pain, you make the least movements possible.

It's like I'm in prison.

Every prison inmate has a movement disorder. Most of the world is out of their reach. They are not able to go where they want to go and do what they want to do.

Their movement disorder they brought on themselves by their actions. They are usually placed in prison because of something they had done.

I don't believe my imprisonment is the result of something I have done. I am in prison none the less. The reason I am not able to do what I want to do and go where I want to go is not because of any crime that I have committed. I guess I'm locked up in this cell of Parkinson's disease because of the crime that was committed by my first parents a long time ago in a garden.

Most prisoners in jail are confined away from the world that was once theirs. They are locked away out of sight. But my prison is right in the middle of my world. That means I can see all the things that are mine, but are now just out of reach.... Picking up my grandson, running, walking normally, doing the work I want to do, having a sex life with my wife, riding a motorcycle, sleeping in my bed. These and innumerable other things that were just a reach away are now just out of reach.

But, I'm not blaming anyone, except the creep that snuck into that garden and offered my first parents a lie. Despite the fact that I will most likely remain in this prison, it is my intention to continue to live a life based on a decision I made when I was 6 years old. That decision was to accept a free gift from God. Based on that decision, one day I will wake up and discover that not only can I reach that pillow, but I can move without pain. I will also realize that the bars of my prison are gone and I am free.

A Strange Question

The story is told.... a man that had a movement disorder for many, many years maintained a spot on the ground next to a pond of water. It was widely known that from time to time, an angel would come by and stir the water. When the angel did this, the first sick person to enter the water was healed. The man could never get to the water fast enough. Someone else always got there before him.
One day Jesus walked up

to the man with the movement disorder and asked him, "Do you want to be well?"

What a strange question to ask a sick person. Of course he wants to be well. I didn't understand why Jesus asked the question until I got Parkinson's.

For a year before I was diagnosed, most of the time I was miserable. I had gone from a very happy, content person to someone that felt depressed and filled with anxiety all the time for no reason. Many years before I started to feel like this, I had gone through two terrible life events that would make anyone feel this way, but that had been long ago. Now life was great with a wonderful wife, three beautiful children, a job I loved, and a beautiful home. Life couldn't have been any better, but I was miserable. I prayed and asked God constantly for relief, but none came. Then things started happening in my body. My left arm stopped swinging when I walked. My left hand would shake when I used it. My left wrist started to hurt. I lost my sense of smell. My voice started to change. I continued to ask God for relief, but none came.

Then one day I went to my doctor for my yearly checkup. Casually, he asked how I was. I told him about the things I was feeling. When I had finished, he looked at me and said," It sounds like you have Parkinson's Disease." I walked out of his office stunned. Then I had a strange feeling, a feeling of relief and happiness. I had been suffering for no reason.... now there was a reason. All of the things that had tormented me turned out to indeed be the symptoms of Parkinson's Disease. A week later, with some new knowledge and some pills, I was my old self again. Yes, it's true I was my old self with Parkinson's, but the suffering had stopped.

Now back to the strange question Jesus asked, "Do you want to be well?"
It's been more than 4 years since I was diagnosed. I started out feeling like my old self, but over time the symptoms have changed and the Parkinson's has progressed. The main way I have been able to live happy with this fact

is to accept it. I try to do all I can to slow the progression, but I know it will continue to progress. For me to deny this would be much more difficult than acceptance. Also, I have been developing defenses to cope with this uninvited intruder. Right or wrong, with acceptance comes familiarity. Although, I fight to keep Parkinson's at bay, it has become one of the things that defines me.

There is a story of a man that spent almost all of his 60 years in prison. One day a parole board told him he was free to go. They opened the prison bars and released him into the free world. He spent the next week trying to find a way to get arrested again. He had come to the place that life behind bars was all he knew.

I don't think I'm saying that if I wake up tomorrow without Parkinson's Disease, I

won't know how to live without it. But I have adjusted to having it. A large part of my acceptance is that even if I am wrong and I am supposed to be healed, God still loves me and is my provider. He will never abandon me.
I do know that if it did go away, something else, maybe even worse, would eventually get me.

One more story;

A group of people were

sitting on the floor in a circle. God told them to throw their biggest problem in life into the middle of the circle. They did. Then he told them they each must choose a problem. They could take any one of them. Each person took their own problem back.

Re: John 5: 1-15 (Bible)

Words And Music

Everything that exists in the physical world is made out of the same stuff, from a butterfly to the universe. Atoms, protons, electrons, neutrons arranged differently to create what they are and do. And what they are and what they do is determined by the laws God set in place to govern their behavior. Everything is not everything. What we can see, hear, touch, taste and smell is just a minor fraction, a microscopic part of what really exists. Everything we can experience through our 5 senses is a mere grain of sand on the beach of reality that is out there within and beyond our universe. Again, we know this because we know this. The fact that we can think and dream and love proves this is true.

Two examples of there being more than everything is music and writing. Both music and writing use a specific number of characters. With music, it's notes and with writing it's the letters of an alphabet. Just as everything in our physical universe was created by God from the same elements, the music that is played is created from the same notes and everything written is from the same letters and ruled by the laws that govern each. Mankind has the mistaken idea that we can be creators. All we can be are assemblers. We can take the things God created and form them into the things we use. We have the raw material and form it into anything the laws that govern that raw material will allow. We take musical notes and arrange them in an order that can be played on an instrument we have constructed from the same material we are made of and play a song. We take the letters of the alphabet and punctuation and write a story.

The ability to do this lets us know that we are more than star stuff. We take letters and form words and arrange the words in an order that when someone reads those words, it changes the readers heart and allows them to understand something they did not understand before. It's magic. Real magic. The same magic that happens when someone takes musical notes and arranges them in such a way that causes a listener to cry. This did not happen by two atoms coming together by themselves and then other atoms coming together over and over until a universe is built. Built by the atoms that it's made of. And these little atoms did this all by themselves? Spontaneously? Without any help? That would be something. That would be like the atoms of a space shuttle deciding to gather together on their own and form a vehicle capable of blasting into space, circling the globe a few times, and then landing safely back on earth.

I like music. I like it because of what it does to me. It makes me happy. It makes me cry. It makes me remember times in my life, both good and bad. When I was falling in love with my wife, the song

"Maniac" from the movie Flashdance would come on the radio and I would think of her. Even now, years later, when I hear that song, I think of her. When my first wife left me, I remember certain songs made me feel that I wasn't alone during this time of heartache and made the pain tolerable. I discovered when the heart is abandoned, it comforts itself by believing that a time will come when the one that abandoned it will regret it. I was drawn to songs like " If the phone doesn't ring, it's me " and " You'll think of me."

I like to listen to music. I don't ever remember wanting to learn the notes and the laws that govern them enough to want to play music. My wife is a classically trained pianist. Not only did she learn the notes and the laws, but she was born with something more than most people are born with. She was born with what's referred to as a gift. It is the extra ability that some people have that goes beyond learning to do something. A gift in music is the ability to not only learn the physical process of playing the notes, but the learning is usually easier for someone gifted. They also are able to express the notes in a way that moves the spirit, soul and body of the ones that hear it. This is not

something that is learned or can even be achieved through practice. I believe it is one of those things that goes beyond the stuff we are made of. It shows us we are more than the sum of our parts.
I think writing is the same way. Everyone, (unless they have a physical or mental challenge that prevents it,) can learn to write. We learn to take the letters of whatever alphabet we know and put them

together applying the laws that govern them and express thoughts. These thoughts can make others laugh, they can teach, establish or change what people believe, share feelings, pass on things that need to be remembered. Words also can be put together to express hatred, tell lies, cause people pain. The greatest thing words can express is love. As with music, I believe people can be gifted in the use of words. They are gifted with the ability to use the same letters everyone uses but put them together in such a way that they speak to the human heart and spirit. I have no idea why some are gifted and some are not. I am sure there are millions of people in the world that are gifted, but they and the ones around them never discover what they have. Millions of people are living in poverty and isolation under oppressive governments having gifting's but never being able to discover or share them.

As I said, I like music. I also like to read. It wasn't until I was a junior in high school that I discovered reading. Up to that time, I had never read a whole book, "except for See Spot Run" in kindergarten. Then, in high school, I was required to take a class in literature. A requirement of the class was to read a book from a list of books. I remember putting the list on my desk, closing my eyes and allowing my finger to drop to the paper and whatever book title my finger landed on, that would be the book I would read. When I opened my eyes, I saw that my finger had chosen "Out of the Silent Planet", by C.S. Lewis. I had never heard of it before and hoped it wouldn't be boring. As I started to read, I found it to be surprisingly interesting. It was about a man on a walking vacation in England being kidnapped and taken to the planet Mars to be sacrificed to the inhabitants. Soon after they landed he was able to escape his kidnappers. He wandered around for a while until he came across a Martian. At first, he was afraid. Then he realized the Martian was not only intelligent, but civilized and even friendly. After some time, he learned to communicate with the Martian.

Then my world changed. It was like being struck by lightning. I discovered the Martians not only knew God, but they knew His son, Jesus. (although they called Him by a different name.)

Being saved at the age of 6, and being a Christian almost all my life and having no interest in reading did limit my exposure somewhat. Going to church a couple times a week, having mostly children's bible stories read to me growing up and then from time to time reading portions of the bible, my experience with other forms of literature was very limited.

But now, at the age of 15 or 16, to be reading a book that was not a bible story or the bible, but it expresses my Christian beliefs in a creative, mature and imaginary way turned out to be life changing for me. I knew I would never be the same.

(The reason the book is titled " Out of the Silent Planet", is because, in the story, it turns out that the entire universe is filled with inhabited planets. They all went through the "serpent and the apple", garden of Eden test. Only one planet failed.... earth. All the other planets chose to do what God asked them to do. This meant that the Martians had a free and open relationship with God and His Son and with all the other planets, except the earth. The earth was a blank spot in the universe and silent.)

That's how I discovered the joy of reading.

Stricken With Parkinson's

The story is told that around 2000 years ago, four men had a friend that had a movement disorder. In the story, it was said the man was stricken with palsy.

The four friends had heard of a man that could heal people was in town. An Old English version of the story describes what happens this way;

(And again, he entered into Capernaum after some days; and it was noised that he was in the house.

And straightway many were gathered together, insomuch that there was no room to receive them, no, not so much as about the door: and he preached the word unto them.

And they come unto him, bringing one sick of the palsy, which was borne of four.

And when they could not come nigh unto him for the press, they uncovered the roof where he was: and when they had broken it up, they let down the bed wherein the sick of the palsy lay.

When Jesus saw their faith, he said unto the sick of the palsy, Son, thy sins be forgiven thee.

But there were certain of

the scribes sitting there, and reasoning in their hearts,

Why doth this man thus speak blasphemies? Who can forgive sins but God only?

And immediately when Jesus perceived in his spirit that they so reasoned within themselves, he said unto them, Why reason ye these things in your hearts?

Whether is it easier to say to the sick of the palsy, Thy sins be forgiven thee; or to say, Arise, and take up thy bed, and walk?

But that ye may know that the Son of man hath power on earth to forgive sins, (he saith to the sick of the palsy,)

I say unto thee, Arise, and take up thy bed, and go thy way into thine house.

And immediately he arose, took up the bed, and went forth before them all; insomuch that they were all amazed, and glorified God.)

These four friends decided to take their friend to this healing man so he would no longer have to live like this. They each grasped a corner of their friend's bed, the bed he had been trapped in for so many years. They carried him to the house where this healing man was. But when they got there, so many people surrounded the house and were blocking the door that they couldn't get close. So, they decided the only way they could get their friend inside was to get on the roof and find a way in from there. Meanwhile, Jesus was inside, talking and healing, when He noticed something falling from the ceiling. He looked up and discovered that someone was making a large hole in the roof. Soon He saw some men were lowering something down to him by ropes tied to the four corners. He stepped back to allow the object to rest on the floor. He saw there was a man on a bed. The man was obviously sick. Jesus looked up again and saw four men with hope shining from their faces looking down at Him through the hole they

had just created.
Jesus then looked at the man on the bed. His entire body from his head to his feet was grossly contorted and continuously shaking. He placed His hand on the man's shoulder. His hand followed the rhythm of the tremors. With compassion and love in His voice, Jesus told him, "Son, your sins are forgiven."
Now earlier, when Jesus had arrived at the house and all the people had

surrounded the doorway, along came a group of the church leaders. The crowd parted to allow the leaders to enter the house.

The moment Jesus told the man his sins were forgiven, the leaders looked at each other and thought to themselves, "He can't say that! Only God can forgive sins." Jesus knew what they were thinking. He turned to the leaders and asked them, "Which one is easier, to tell this poor man his sins are forgiven, or to tell him to get up and walk? I will show you that I have the power to do both." With that, Jesus turned back to the man lying on the bed, His hand still moving in time with the tremors. He looked at him and said, " Get up and pick up your bed and go home."

Immediately, Jesus hand and the man's body became perfectly still. Jesus stepped back.

Every eye was on the man on the bed. Slowly, he started to move, but these were not involuntary movements they had witnessed for so long. These were slow, deliberate movements. It was like watching the birth of a butterfly. As he got up, he transformed from a curled up, contorted, shaking figure into a normal man, standing straight and tall. He stood there for a moment or two, looking around at all the amazed faces, (except for the stone faces of the church leaders, who were obviously not sharing in everyone else's joy). He looked up through the hole in the roof at his four friends. How could he ever thank them? Lastly, He looked over at Jesus. He couldn't seem to find any words. Jesus just smiled and tilted His head to the side as if to say, "Go home."

The man bent down, picked up his bed and

left the house, a free man.

(The definition of palsy is:

pal·sy
ˈpôlzē/
noundated
1.
paralysis, especially that which is accompanied by involuntary tremors.
"a kind of palsy had seized him"
verb

1.
affect with paralysis and involuntary tremors. "she feels as if the muscles on her face are palsied")

In 1817, a London doctor named James Parkinson wrote a paper describing people that had difficulty with movement along with uncontrolled tremors. He named the condition, "The Shaky Palsy". Soon after he published his article, it began to be called

Parkinson's disease.)
Re: Luke: 5: 17-26
(Bible)

Not For A Lack Of Stones

When we were first married, my husband and I spent most of our time together. As the years went by, he seemed to be away from home more and more. He was away from our village much of the time. I was lonely.

I had become friends with a man that sold eggs at the market. I found myself going to the market often. Each time I would pass by his egg stand, we would talk. He was always very pleasant and funny. He seemed to understand me. I found I was becoming attracted to him. Our talks made me less lonely.

One night when my husband was away, there was a knock at my door. It was my friend from the market. He asked if he could come in so we could talk for a while. I said yes. I poured some wine and we sat at the table and we started to talk. We had spoken enough in the past that we knew each other's stories and troubles. As I talked again about my loneliness, he placed his hand on mine. It was the first time we had ever touched. He picked up my hand and softly kissed it. I kissed his in return. One thing led to another and soon we were in my bed.

Suddenly, the door to my house flew open with a terrible crash. I felt many strong hands grabbing my legs and pulling me out my door. I was pulled out into the street, my hand grasping my blanket. All I could hear were angry voices and all I could feel was the pain and helplessness and humiliation of being dragged naked through the streets. Finally, we came to a stop. I struggled to raise my head and look around to discover what was happening to me.

We were in a small courtyard. All around me were the angry faces of the leaders of my village. I rose to my knees and wrapped my blanket around me to try to cover up a small part of my shame. The village leaders kept pointing and shouting at me. Slowly, they stopped shouting and it became very quiet. I then noticed another group of men, separate from the men that had dragged me here. One of our leaders began to speak to them. He said," This woman, (pointing his finger at me), was caught in the act of adultery. The Scriptures say she must be stoned to death. What do you say?"

One of the men he was speaking to bent down and began writing on the ground. After a while he stood up and said, "The one among you that has never sinned, you throw the first stone." Then he bent back down and continued writing.

I lowered my head, shaking uncontrollably. I hugged my legs as tight as I could, waiting for the first stone to strike me. I wondered how many stones would have to hit me before I died. I thought about how painful it will be and how long the pain would last. I also thought about the shame of how I would be remembered.

It felt like an eternity had passed by, but nothing happened. I kept my eyes closed. The only sound I finally heard sounded like stones hitting the ground and footsteps fading away.

When I gathered enough courage to look up, I found I was there all alone, except for the man that had been writing on the ground. He asked me, "Do you see any of the men who were condemning you?" I answered, "No". Then he said," I don't condemn you either. You are free. Go and don't sin anymore".

Re: John 8:2-11 (Bible)

Cries From Heaven

I was on vacation on Sanibel Island. This was the third consecutive year my two best friends and I had driven from Orlando to this island we had grown to love. The plan was to get away from our normal lives for a week. The three of us worked as veterinary techs at three different animal clinics. All of us were born in the same year and at the same hospital, Orlando Regional. Despite living in the same city and doing the same work, we had never run into each other. We had attended different high schools. We met one Saturday shopping at the Mall at Millenia. We were each searching for the perfect swimsuit and have been best friends ever since. The fact that we worked for different animal hospitals made it possible for us to take the same week off each year and vacation together.

This year we rented a condo for a week at the Oceans Reach Resort. We made this choice because we discovered in our search for the perfect place to spend our vacation, the Oceans Reach was the closest condo complex to the beach we could find.

Vacationing together had many advantages for three single young girls. Cost savings, of course. We would also watch out for each other for protection (safety in numbers). We would watch over each other when it came to guys. Three girls on vacation on a tropical island is to guys like blood in the water is to a shark. So, we protected each other from making relational mistakes. We set rules for ourselves. No guys in the condo. No single dates. All for one and one for all. That meant even if only one of us had a date, the other two would also go on the date. We would always stay together, no matter what. We very quickly discovered that there were always enough guys to go around, so no one ever had to go along on a date alone.

Each year we would make sure to eat at all our favorite restaurants. One called The Bubble Room is at the top of the list. They always had great food, a fun atmosphere, and huge slices of cake we would purchase to take back to the condo for dessert later in the evening. This year it was just as good. And as usual, when we arrived, it wasn't very long before the sharks started circling.

Of course, meeting guys and enjoying their company was a big part of our vacation adventure each year. The sharks circling was something we looked forward to. If it didn't happen, we would be disappointed. It was fun to be three young women in this tropical paradise. We would play the usual games to size up the sharks and decide if they were worthy of us.

Then, out of the corner of my eye, I saw Jon.

We were sitting at our table eating our food when I noticed him. He was breathtaking... sun-bleached long blond hair, a deep bronze tan and a chiseled body. He was wearing a white button-down shirt, untucked and spotless. He had on a pair of classy looking jeans with just the right tightness to reveal the strong muscles of his perfectly shaped legs. On his feet were flip flops that had seen a good number of miles. There were two guys with him and they were walking directly towards us. As they came closer, my friends and I prepared ourselves. But the unexpected happened. They passed right by us without a sign of knowing we were even there. We were surprised and slightly insulted.

The boys stopped at the corner pool table and started to play a game. My friends and I got over the obvious rejection and turned our attention back to our grouper sandwiches and cold slaw.

A short time later, we got that shark bait feeling again. There were two other guys approaching our table and this time it was apparent that we were the target. We noticed these two earlier because of a disruption they had caused with two other girls. They were loud and slightly drunk then, and unfortunately for us, had been drinking ever since. It was obvious that now they were very drunk. When they arrived at our table, they immediately began making rude, loud comments along with suggestions that we go with them to "really have some fun". As they started to pull on us to get us to go with them, I heard a strong clear voice come from behind me. "It looks to me like these nice girls don't want to go with you." I turned and looked past the man that had my arm to see whose voice it was, and saw it belonged to Jon. I guess when our assault began, Jon and his friends put down their cue sticks and followed the noise. Now the two guys that were trying to force us to leave had three guys behind them. I heard Jon's voice again. "I suggest you take your hands off them," he said. One of the men replied, "I suggest you mind your own business". Almost immediately, I felt the hold on my arm loosen and I heard what sounded like choking. A second later, I was free. I turned to find the guy that was pulling on me in the firm embrace of Jon. Jon had a choke hold on the guy's neck and was pulling him to the exit. The guy's face was turning colors as they went. They were closely followed by the other one being carried by Jon's two companions. One had the creep by the feet, and the other was carrying him under his armpits. There was a stream of blood flowing from the second man's nose.

After a few minutes, Jon and his two buddies returned to the restaurant and this time walked straight to our table. We quickly realized they had saved us. They assured us we would not be bothered by those two again. We invited them to join us. They sat down and after the introductions, we began to get to know each other. Almost immediately, the conversations split up into twos. Jon started to direct his conversation to me. He asked the normal get to know you questions and I answered them. Then it was my turn to ask him questions.

He told me that the three of them had met 3 days ago on a beach on

Captiva, an island just to the north of Sanibel. The two islands are connected by a small bridge. Actually, they did not meet on the beach but about 200 ft off the beach, in the Gulf of Mexico. They had arrived at the beach at around the same time, but separately. They each had a surf board and had pushed off into the water. They noticed each other 150 ft out and had stopped together about

200 ft from the shore. All three had the same puzzled look on their face. The water was completely calm. Not even a ripple. No one had told them that the Gulf was usually not the best place to surf. They realized that must be why they were the only ones along the whole beach that were on surf boards. They sat there, side by side like chess pieces. Floating almost motionless, waiting for

the wave that would never come. Finally, they looked at each other, sweat dripping off their chins. Without saying a word, all three rolled off their boards into the cool water and then remounted the boards and paddled in to shore.

When they got to the beach, they sat down under some trees and talked for a while. They discovered they were staying at the same resort. All three were single and unattached. They decided to change clothes and meet at the resorts tennis courts, play a few games and then meet for dinner that night. That's why they were at the Bubble Room. That's why they were available to save us.

After we finished our meals and bought our

slices of cake, the six of us stood out in the parking lot for a while talking. One of Jon's friends asked if we would all like to go to his condo to eat cake and watch a movie? We girls excused ourselves for a minute to talk. When we were far enough away from the boys not to be overheard and asked each other what we thought. We quickly decided because we would be together and they seemed nice, we would accept their invitation. It was 8:00, so we said we would stay until midnight.

We got in our car and they got in theirs and we followed them to the South Seas Resort, just up the road from the restaurant. The resort was beautiful and the condo faced the Gulf.

 We decided we were all too full from dinner to

eat cake, so we agreed to watch the movie first and have cake later. After looking over the DVD choices, we chose the old classic, The Wizard of Oz. As we found our places to get comfortable to watch the movie, we paired up like it had been since the restaurant. It was Jon and me on the love seat and the other two couples on the couch. As the movie started, Jon sat close to me. Just about the time the Scarecrow and Dorothy meet, I felt Jon take my hand. He took it slowly and gently, probably so I wouldn't be startled and pull away. I didn't. We sat there, slouched and holding hands for the rest of the movie. When the credits started to roll at the end of the movie, all three guys got up and said they were going to serve the cake. This was turning out to be a great evening. The three of them went into the kitchen and about a minute later, Jon came back out with an ice bucket in his hand. He asked me if I would go with him downstairs to the ice machine. I said "sure". As we walked down the stairs, he reached for my hand and I laced my fingers with his. When we reached the first-floor ice machine, we both gasped at the same time. Over the horizon of the gulf was the most beautiful moon I had ever seen rising above the horizon. Jon asked me if I would like to step out onto the beach to get a better look? I said yes.

We walked down a short path through some palms and palmetto bushes and came out onto a completely deserted beach. The moon and the ocean were breathtaking. Soft gentle waves rippled lazily onto the sand. We walked down to the water's edge, my fingers still laced in his. I looked back towards the buildings and could see the lights of the resort shining through the palms. Jon asked if I wanted to sit for a few minutes. I again said yes. We sat there for three or four minutes enjoying the moonrise and the breeze from the gulf. I felt his hand release mine. Then I could feel his hand softly rest on the small of my back and slowly rise until his fingers were tangled in my hair. I turned to look into his eyes. But instead of the soft blue I had seen all evening, I saw something dark. Suddenly, his hand grabbed my hair and he pulled my head back violently. Instead of his pleasant voice, I heard an evil voice say, "Now let's have some fun." I tried to scream but he clamped his other hand over my mouth and nose. I was having trouble breathing. I tried to break free but he was too strong. In one motion, he pushed me all the way back and rolled on top of me. His legs were holding my arms down as he sat on my stomach. He continued to hold one hand over my mouth and nose and with the other, held my head down. I couldn't breathe. I kept fighting and trying to scream until everything went black.

I awoke to the smell of garbage. My whole body ached, especially my head and the left side of my face. As my eyes started to focus, I realized it was dark. It was night. I was in some kind of small room with no roof and a big blue box in front of me... It was a dumpster! I was laying on the dirty concrete floor of a dumpster enclosure. I tried to remember how I got here but I had no idea. The last thing I remembered was being held down by Jon. What had he done to me? Why was I here? Where are my friends? With great pain, I slowly got up. I could see from the light of a streetlamp that my shirt was badly torn and my shorts and swim suit bottoms were gone. I carefully squeezed passed the smelly dumpster and looked around. It appeared that I was behind a restaurant. There were some full length white cook's aprons hung up on some nails on the back of the building. I took two down to cover myself, one in the front and one for the back. I looked at my watch. It said 4:17. I slowly walked around to the front of the restaurant. I saw the sign, R.C. Otters. At 4 am, the restaurant and streets were deserted. I started walking. The street was lined with vacation rentals. I walked along, looking back and forth until I saw a house with a light on inside. I could see through the window an older lady sitting in a chair, reading. I approached the door and knocked. I heard footsteps come to the door and a lady's voice ask,

"Who is it?" I answered, "My name is Crystal Wells. I've been hurt and I need help." She said,

"Just a minute." I heard footsteps walk away from the door and then some muffled voices. The door opened and standing there was the lady I had seen through the window and a sleepy looking older man. One look at me and the woman said, "Oh my poor dear!" She took me by the hand and led me to the kitchen and sat me down. While they introduced themselves to me, she got a clean dish towel, wet it, and started to clean my face and cuts. I heard the man, her husband it turned out, talking to someone on the phone. When he had hung up, he came over and told me the police were on their way.

When they arrived, a woman police officer sat with me asking me questions. I told her all I could remember. She then told me that hours ago my friends had reported me missing and they had been searching for me ever since. A short time later, my friends arrived, and after a tearful reunion, the police took all of our statements. The paramedics were there to examine me and care for my injuries. They asked if I had been raped. I said no. I'm not sure why I said that, because I really had no idea if I had been or not, blacking out like I did. The thought of going through some kind of exam after all that had happened to me seemed too embarrassing to endure.

The next two days were spent with the police trying to find out what had happened. We managed to find our way back to the condo where we had watched the movie. We found two of the guys there, but no Jon. They said they had never heard of a Jon. They held to the story that the two of them had picked up my two friends at the Bubble

Room that night and ended up at the condo to watch the Wizard of Oz until the two girls left at midnight. They had never seen me before and didn't know anything about a Jon person. So, after all the questions and investigation, we didn't have any idea what happened....and Jon was a ghost.

When the three of us got home, we spoke a few times but something had changed. I had changed. My two friends just became reminders of that horrible night. I found myself getting angry and isolated. I went back to my job and my life, but there was no joy in anything anymore.

After a month back home, I started getting sick in the morning. Every day I felt sick.

Then I realized I had missed my period. I purchased a home test from the drug store. Standing in my bathroom, staring at the result on the plastic stick, I realized the life I had dreamed of living had just ended. I was pregnant. For a week after finding out, I called in sick at work and never left my apartment. I didn't want to be a mother. A single mother. The mother of a child whose father beat and abused and raped me. I was angry. I hated the man that did this to me. I was angry at my friends that had failed me. I was angry at God for letting this happen to me. I was mad at myself for putting myself in the situation that allowed it to happen. I wasn't going to be forced into a life situation I didn't want or ask for or deserve.

The next Monday I started my research on how I was going to free myself from this. I made an appointment at Planned Parenthood. I heard they helped women free themselves from this problem. I talked with two women, filled out some paperwork and made the appointment for the procedure.

The day arrived and I was ready to get this out of the way and get on with the life I had planned. When I stepped out of my car at the clinic, I noticed some people on the sidewalk in front of the building. They were carrying signs. It looked like they were protesting about something. I didn't pay any attention to them and walked to the entrance of the clinic.

I entered the building and after a few minutes in the waiting area, I was ushered back to a room. They asked me to remove my clothes and put on the gown that they provided for me. A nurse came into the room and asked me to lay on the table that was in the middle of the room and put my feet in the stirrups. I was laying there trying to relax as much as I could when the doctor came in. He told me I had nothing to worry about and this would be over before I knew it. As he started, I was feeling discomfort.

Halfway through the procedure, I started to hear a baby cry. I asked the people in the room, "Why is that baby crying?" They listened and then the nurse standing next to the doctor said,

" There are no babies crying here." She told me it was probably just my imagination and to ignore it.

After a while, the doctor was finished. He stood, removed his gloves and left the room. As I got dressed and got ready to leave, I could still hear the cry. As I walked through the building to go home, I kept looking around to see if I could tell where the crying was coming from. When I went outside to get in my car, I again noticed the people on the sidewalk carrying the protest signs. I decided to walk towards them to see if one of them had a crying baby. No one did. What I did discover was that the signs they were holding had words on them like abortion and choice. And to my horror, the signs also had photos of what appeared to be tiny dismembered arms and legs. A frozen chill went up my spine and I felt like I was going to throw-up. These photos couldn't be real. What they had just done inside that building was remove a glob of tissue. Not a baby. When I saw a woman coming from the group walking towards me, I quickly turned and headed to the parking lot as fast as I could.

When I closed the door to my car, I could no longer hear the crying baby. But I had a very strange feeling. It felt like when my dad died 5 years before. Leaving the memorial service, I felt an emptiness I had never felt before. It was like the world was suddenly empty. Now...the world feels even emptier.

I drove home and that night, I was awakened from a sound sleep. Somewhere, there was a baby crying. I tried putting my pillow over my head to stop me from hearing the cry, but nothing worked. What was strange was that it sounded like the same baby I heard at the planned parenthood building. Wouldn't all baby cries sound the same to me? But this cry sounded different than other cries I had heard.

As the days went by, every few days I would hear that baby, but not always crying. Sometimes laughing, sometimes gurgling like babies do. After a while, even though sometimes the baby would wake me in the middle of the night, I slowly got used to hearing it. As time went by, the baby's voice changed. It was like she was getting older. I say she because it was obvious when she got old enough, I was hearing the voice of a little girl. I got so used to her being there, I decided to give her a name. I chose Coral.

When she started to say words, they were of a language I had never heard and did not understand. Regardless, sometimes it felt like we were having a conversation, even though I had no idea what she was saying.

Seven years went by. Life had found a new normal. I had finished college and started a new career. The days passed, one by one, and my life became what I would call ordinary...except for the fact that the world continued to feel empty, and I had an ongoing conversation with a young girl I couldn't see.

One day, I was looking for a book to read at Barnes & Noble. I found a book called The Message and decided to buy it. When I got home, I discovered it was a bible. I hadn't read the bible since Sunday School when I was 7. Out of curiosity, I opened it up and read a couple of pages. This bible was different than the one I remembered from childhood. There were no thee's or thou's. The words seemed familiar and even a little comforting. So, I continued to read. I found I understood this bible. It almost felt as though the words were written to me. I continued to read. Every morning I would read a little more.

Ever since that horrible night on Captiva Island, I would regularly dream about the events of that night. Many times, that night would invade my waking thoughts as well. Whenever my mind would take me back there, I found I could easily renew my hatred for Jon. I would also renew my anger for those I felt let me down. This renewal was something that became very familiar to me. It seemed as though I needed to keep those feelings close to me, especially my hatred of Jon.

Then one day, my mind went back to that night like it had so many times before. This time though, something was different. Something had changed. I thought back to the beach and Jon, but the hatred was gone. I remembered the story I had read that morning in the bible about Jesus hanging up on that wooden cross, nailed there with spikes. As he looked down at the people that had done this to him, He said to his father, "Forgive them, because they don't know what they are doing." Forgive...the word echoed in my head. Is that what is different? Have I forgiven Jon? The moment I had the thought, I knew it was true. But didn't I need to hold onto the hatred? I couldn't think of a reason I needed too. A deep feeling of release and freedom vibrated through me. I dreamt about the Captiva events the next night, but instead of waking up full of hatred and resentment, I felt joy.

Life was much happier after that. But the world still felt empty

For some reason, the date I went to planned parenthood and had the procedure has stuck in my mind. October 16th. Today it was 12 years ago. This morning, I was in my living room reading my bible, when suddenly everything went dark. After a few moments of fear and concern, it was light again. Except now, I wasn't in my living room anymore. I was at the edge of a forest facing a green field with a sparkling, blue pond in the center of the field. It was a clear fresh morning. I noticed a young girl playing at the edge of the water. I saw a man sitting on a rock a short distance away. He appeared to be watching over her. He motioned for me to come over to where he was and patted his hand on the rock inviting me to sit next to him. I walked over and sat down. He said hello. I said hi. Then he looked over at the girl on the beach. She was making a sand castle. He said, "Isn't she beautiful?" I looked over to where the little girl was playing and as I was about to answer him, she turned, looked at me and smiled. I fell to my knees. Tears filled my eyes. I began to sob. I knew the moment she looked at me, she was my daughter. The baby I had aborted 12 years ago.

She ran up to me and threw her arms around my neck. She whispered "mommy" softly in my ear with the same voice I had heard the last 12 years. I cupped her face in my hands and kissed her cheeks until they were red. I looked into her beautiful blue eyes and said," I love you." She looked back at me and said, "I love you, mommy." I hugged her so tight. Suddenly, she got up and ran towards the forest. I then noticed at the edge of the trees stood a group of children about her age. When she reached them, she turned, smiled and waved. Then they all disappeared into the forest.

I turned to the man, my eyes still filled with tears. I was unable to speak. He reached out his hands to hold mine and said, " We will take good care of her until you return." He then let go of my hands. As he did, I noticed that his hands were scarred. I was about to ask him when I could come back when everything went dark again. After a few moments, I was back in my living room.

The next few days were full of emotions. Sadness for what I had missed and was missing. Happiness knowing my daughter was well and I would see her again.

.....And the world didn't feel empty anymore.

www.ingramcontent.com/pod-product-compliance
Lightning Source LLC
Chambersburg PA
CBHW050150230526
45470CB00001B/40